**Penguin Books**

**The Well Woman Handbook**

Suzie Hayman trained as a teacher at Newcastle University. In 1975 she joined the Family Planning Association as press assistant, subsequently becoming press officer. She was information officer for Brook Advisory Centres from 1976 to 1984 and since then has been a freelance journalist and broadcaster. Suzie Hayman has written for national magazines such as *Woman*, *Woman and Home*, *Living*, *Good Housekeeping*, *Just 17*, *19* and *Country Living*, as well as for the *Guardian* and *Sunday Times* newspapers, and is 'agony aunt' for *Essentials* magazine. She has produced educational material for the Family Planning Association, and is the author of *Hysterectomy*, *It's more than sex: a survival guide to the teenage years* and *Living with a teenager*. A frequent contributor to television and radio, she currently writes and presents the weekly feature *What's the problem?* for Border TV. She lives in Cumbria with her partner and two cats.

D1495501

SUZIE HAYMAN

# *The*
# *Well Woman*
# *Handbook*

ILLUSTRATED BY AUDREY BESTERMAN

PENGUIN BOOKS

PENGUIN BOOKS
Published by the Penguin Group
27 Wrights Lane, London w8 5tz, England
Viking Penguin Inc., 40 West 23rd Street, New York, New York 10010, USA
Penguin Books Australia Ltd, Ringwood, Victoria, Australia
Penguin Books Canada Ltd, 2801 John Street, Markham, Ontario, Canada, l3r 1b4
Penguin Books (NZ) Ltd, 182–190 Wairau Road, Auckland 10, New Zealand

Penguin Books Ltd, Registered Offices: Harmondsworth, Middlesex, England

First published 1989
10 9 8 7 6 5 4 3 2 1

Copyright © Suzie Hayman, 1989
Illustrations copyright © Audrey Besterman, 1989
All rights reserved
Photograph © Carole Easton

Made and printed in Great Britain by Richard Clay Ltd, Bungay, Suffolk
Filmset in Monophoto Photina

# Contents

## Chapter 6: CONTRACEPTION

## Chapter 7: WHERE DO YOU GO?

## Chapter 8: QUESTIONS AND ANSWERS

# Acknowledgements

I would like to thank Toni Belfield, for her help and many invaluable suggestions; Fay Hutchinson, for twelve years' training (and it isn't over yet, my dear. I intend getting my full Smith Haut-Lafitte's worth!); and My Old Man, the best Well Woman Care *I* know (and the typing's terrific, too).

# Introduction

Most of us who own a car will recognize that we cannot expect it to run, day in and day out, without some form of maintenance and care. Not only should we give it the proper fuel and protect it from corrosion, we need to check quite regularly that all the working parts are in good order. We know that identifying a worn tyre or dirty plug *before* its condition worsens is cheaper and less dangerous than waiting until a major repair is necessary. Why then do most of us neglect the vehicle that *all* of us use every day – our own body?

Bodies can break down and develop faults and it often appears that women's bodies are particularly prone to this. However, in spite of appearances, women are far from being the weaker sex. Given equal care and attention, a girl baby has a greater chance of survival than a boy, and women have a longer life expectancy. Women may have less strength than men, but they have greater stamina and resistance to disease. But women also tend to be neglected, both by those around them and by themselves, and to come under greater strains than men. In the past twenty years, the number of women entering the labour market in the UK has increased so that women make up some 40 per cent of the work-force. Yet there is no evidence to suggest that men are increasing their share of domestic or child-care duties proportionally. So most women carry a double or even triple burden, working both in and outside the home. Their well-being often suffers as a result.

In spite of this, women – even more than men – tend to neglect their health. It can be hard to recognize or believe how much influence we have over our own well-being. We care about our appearance and often spend time, money, effort and concern on how we look. Part of this may involve us in studying our bodies from day to day and worrying about or even changing our behaviour to improve matters. But, much of the time, it is only the superficial aspects we try to control. Ironically, the healthier you are, the better you feel and the better you look. These three factors tend to go together.

The running checks we keep on ourselves already could be of far greater use to us. What most of us need to do to improve our lives enormously is to widen the scope of these checks. They can become part of a whole range of systematic care that helps you live a longer, happier, healthier life. It only takes the understanding that you can have a surprisingly significant effect on yourself to give you the motivation, and a bit of information to give you the confidence to start.

We can all grow up with startling gaps in our knowledge about ourselves, particularly about the parts of our bodies that we often refer to as our 'private parts'. Every year, thousands of women suffer from infections or diseases of the reproductive organs, ranging from irritating or debilitating to the downright dangerous, rather than go to a doctor for advice. For it is doctors or other health professionals that we see as the sources of help, not ourselves. 22,000 women every year even die from cancer of the cervix, ovary and breast. Yet in many cases these conditions could be easily detected, treated and often cured – if only women had the knowledge to know that something was wrong, that something could be done, and the confidence to demand that action be taken. It could be argued that for many of these women, fear and lack of information disable and kill, more than the diseases themselves.

Women are often shut off from health care by a complex series of barriers. The most obvious one is the lack of time many of us have in which to look after ourselves. Women are the nurturers in our society – we run homes, bring up children, care for our partners – and we are brought up to think that this is where we gain our value and status. A woman who takes time out to care for herself will often feel she is being 'selfish', since this appears to rob the people she 'should' be looking after of her time and attention. Women who work outside the home will have even less time to spare, and may already feel guilty at not always being available to their families. Even women without families will still feel that spending time on themselves is somehow vain or inconsiderate. It is not so much that there is little time to spare – it is the belief that any free time should be spent on 'important' concerns, and women and their health are not considered important.

Women are not the only ones to have this conviction. Many women who ask for help from agony aunts explain their reluctance to go to their own doctors by saying, 'He always makes me feel that I am wasting his time.' They may be projecting their own guilt on to the doctor, but equally there are still male doctors who are inclined to dismiss the worries of their women patients as being trivial, neurotic . . . 'female'.

A further barrier is erected by ignorance. We still suffer from the lingering conviction that certain parts of our bodies are taboo and not to be touched or looked at by ourselves, or shown to other people. In spite of the apparent high profile of sexual information in our society, we are in fact remarkably unwilling to talk openly about the subject. Sex and sexuality are constantly referred to by innuendo, but honest and clear discussion is shunned and suppressed. The result is often that, while we may go to a pharmacist for treatment for a pain in a limb, or to a doctor for advice on ulcers in the mouth, if the area concerned is anywhere near vulva or breasts we shy away from disclosure. These areas can be seen as 'dirty', and an infection in them may bring down an accusation of immoral behaviour. As an agony aunt, I am constantly receiving letters from girls and women who have problems, often of long duration and extreme discomfort, who insist, 'Don't tell me to go to my doctor because I would be far too embarrassed.' Secrecy and shame also make many of us feel particularly vulnerable, so the threat of a disease in our sexual parts is seen as a threat to our sexuality. Most of us suffer from the ostrich syndrome – ignore it and it will go away! Furthermore, deep-seated and superstitious fears are attached to the naming of a problem. Somehow, the feeling is, if the lump is not *called* cancer, it will not *be* cancer. The less we know about ourselves, the easier it is to surrender to such fears.

A third barrier is the impression that all health care is doctor and 'ill-person' orientated. We see health care as a situation where we take steps only when symptoms of an illness have developed and then the step we take is to approach the appropriate specialist – a doctor, a dentist, a chiropodist. Having done so, we put ourselves in their hands and allow them to make a diagnosis, decide on the treatment and cure us. If we accept this view, we see certain parts of our bodies as being 'off-limits' to ourselves, not to be tampered with by our hands but as the territory of the doctor or nurse. We also see certain information in the same light, not to be dabbled with by non-professionals and to be kept as the exclusive property of those in whom we put our trust.

The concept of Well Woman care challenges all these views. Well Woman care is preventative. It encourages women, and the professionals to whom they may turn, to invest their efforts in maintaining good health instead of having to deal with bad. Health is not just a matter of absence of disease or a swift cure for an illness. Being healthy is a positive state. Well Woman care puts the responsibility for our health back into our own hands, where it belongs and where it is best conducted. Instead of being a helpless patient who gives her health into the hands of doctors, we can take on ourselves the responsibility for our own care, taking steps to ensure our day-to-day activities and behaviour give us a greater chance of staying well.

Well Woman care is 'holistic'. That is, it recognizes that for any particular part of your body to remain healthy, the *whole* body must be functioning as well as it can. And for this to be possible, you need to consider your entire lifestyle – your diet, your work, your leisure, your relationships and your environment. The more we know about our bodies and how they work, and how our sex lives, working lives and leisure lives can affect us, the better opportunities we have to make these effects good ones. Well Woman care encourages women to make some health checks for themselves and to learn when some conditions would be responsive to self-help and not necessarily need the intervention of a doctor. Well Woman care also encourages women to examine and get to know their bodies well enough to recognize when a problem needs to be investigated by a professional adviser.

Well Woman care recognizes that women need to look after themselves, if for no other reason than to allow themselves to be better carers of their families. A worried, ailing mother is hardly likely to be able to give better attention to her partner and children than a confident and fit one. More important to many people is the fact that women have as much responsibility to themselves as to others, and have the right to put their own well-being on an equal or more prominent footing. Preventative care is also far more efficient – and less expensive – than care offered after the event. By looking for and recognizing the early signs of irritating or harmful conditions, women and their advisers can forestall or treat problems that might otherwise prove awkward, long-lasting or even fatal.

To do this, we need information, and that is what this book is all about. It is not intended as a replacement for a doctor's help or advice. You will not be able to learn how to diagnose or treat major illness from one slim volume! However, *The Well Woman Handbook* will enable you to learn about your body and to accept that every part of it *is* yours, and not the exclusive preserve of your doctors. In it we shall be giving hints on how to care for yourself; how to maintain your health; how to tell when some aspect might give you cause for concern; how to approach professionals for their help in your efforts and what to expect when you do so. In effect, it is a service manual for your body throughout its life, and one that you can pass on to your friends, neighbours, daughters and mothers, and indeed to the men in your life.

Well Woman care is 'empowering'; not only does it give us responsibility for our lives, it gives us far more control. Some people fear that 'a little learning is a dangerous thing'. The original author of this – Alexander Pope – could not have agreed more, but not in the way his statement is usually quoted to mean. It is only incomplete or insufficient knowledge that is harmful, while a fuller understanding protects and enables. I hope after reading the Handbook you will feel far more knowledgeable about yourself, your body, your choices and your rights, and be able to remain a Well Woman!

# CHAPTER 1

# *The Female Body –*
# *How it Works When*
# *All is Well*

We take it for granted that faces, like fingerprints, are all different. We share common features – noses, mouths and eyes – and they tend to be arranged in roughly the same order. But the subtleties of shape and size make each of us separate individuals. Bodies, both externally and internally, are equally individual. We all have the same parts, but their size, shape, colour and texture will be slightly different in each of us. This chapter will describe the likely appearance of your body, how it functions when all is well, and how it is likely to change during your normal monthly cycle and throughout your life. However, to a certain extent this can be only a guide. The information needs to be interpreted and applied by you to your own self and experience.

The range of what is 'normal' for individual women can be enormous and it is very unwise for one woman to compare herself to another and to feel either of them is unusual, freakish, less feminine or sexually inadequate because a difference emerges. Comparison *can* be helpful, however, if it helps us to recognize the diversity of our bodies and to feel more comfortable in looking at and discussing them. The aim of a guide such as this is not to set up a standard to which the reader must try to conform, but to help you learn what is normal for *you*. When you can do this, you can judge for yourself which discharges and odours, lumps, bumps or twiddly bits are natural and which should prompt action or a request for further advice.

We may inherit tendencies towards developing certain illnesses but there is no doubt that our lifestyle – our sexual, social, dietary and working habits and the ways we do or do not look after ourselves – has enormous influence on our health. For us to know how we can shape these influences we need to understand how our bodies work. The function of any living being is to survive and reproduce itself. Very few women in Western society have as many offspring as our bodies are capable of bearing. However, our reproductive system is geared to produce young, and our hormonal system prompts us to do so. Being 'natural', that is being sexually active and producing children, puts women at a higher risk of certain reproductive disorders – such as prolapse of the uterus and cancer of the cervix – than being celibate and childless. Not using the equipment as nature intended carries its own risks, however. Nuns have a higher risk of breast cancer than mothers! Why this is so will be discussed later.

As women, we pass through three main stages in our lives and our bodies alter in each of these. Around 16 per cent of our lives is spent as pre-pubertal children. A transitional period lasting several years then carries us into the fertile portion of our lives. This is followed by another five to ten years of transition which leads us into the third or quarter of our lives during which we are post-menopausal. In each of these stages, our bodies look and function differently, and in our fertile period they also alter during each menstrual cycle.

The organs and parts of the body that make up a woman's reproductive system and that we shall be looking at in detail are: the vulva, clitoris, cervix and uterus, fallopian tubes, ovaries, hypothalamus and pituitary glands and the breasts. The rectum and anus, bladder and urethra are related organs and they also need to be discussed when considering this area.

A woman's femininity lies, not in the size or shape of her sexual organs, but in how she feels about herself. Her gender is decided from the moment of conception although, curiously enough, both male and female foetuses develop along identical lines until around the eighth week of growth. At this point, organs which would become testicles and penis in a male child become ovaries and clitoris in a female child. A woman is still a woman, however, even when she is not exercising her body's potential. You are female before you mature and become capable of being pregnant, and after you have aged beyond the stage of having children. You are female if you are unable to have children, or if you choose not to do so. You are female if you choose not to have heterosexual sex or if you choose not to have sex at all.

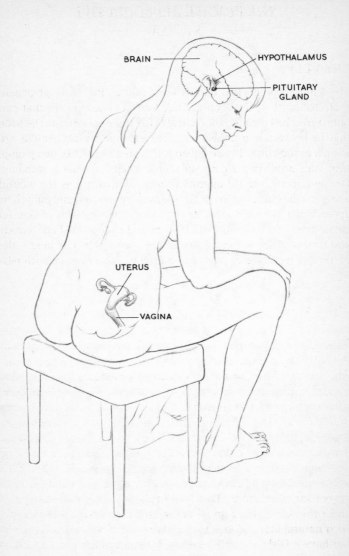

BRAIN

HYPOTHALAMUS

PITUITARY GLAND

UTERUS

VAGINA

The location of the hypothalamus, pituitary gland and the pelvic reproductive organs

# THE FEMALE REPRODUCTIVE
## ——— SYSTEM ———

### THE VULVA

The female reproductive organs are found in the lower abdomen, protected by the pelvic bones. They form a closed system that can only be reached through the central of the three openings to the body that lie between a woman's legs. The external female genitals are known as the vulva. Before puberty, this area consists of two plump, neat folds divided by a deep slit visible when the child is standing. During puberty, the slit appears to move downward as the mound above it – the mons veneris or Hill of Love – rounds out and pubic hair appears and hides the area. At the same time, the folds of skin on either side of the openings will thicken and change in shape, colour and texture. They surround two of the openings in this area – the urethra or waste-water passage, and the vagina or sex or birth passage.

### THE LABIA

These fleshy folds are called labia – the Greek word for 'lips'. The inner pair or labia minora (small lips) often turn a darker colour than the outer lips and are hairless and shiny. Labia often appear somewhat coarse in texture and frilly or wrinkled at the edges. The labia minora are often smaller in size than the enfolding labia majora, although quite a few women find they do actually hang down lower than the outer folds. The outer sides of the labia majora are usually covered in hair. Both sets can be small and neat or long and pendulous, hanging down quite a way. Labia are often asymmetrical, with one side being plumper or longer than the other.

The surface of the labia minora and the inner surface of the labia majora are often moist. This is the result of the sebaceous glands under the skin exuding an oil to keep the area flexible and healthy. Such natural lubrication is by no means 'dirty' although at times it can have a fairly distinctive odour. This part of the body is rich in apocrine or sweat glands which can manufacture a natural scent, the function of which is to attract the attention of a member of the opposite sex. In a society that places an unnatural value on being

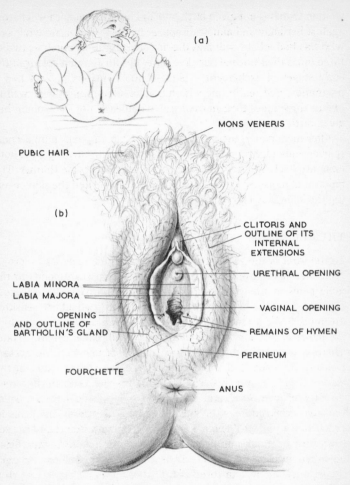

(a)

MONS VENERIS

PUBIC HAIR

(b)

CLITORIS AND OUTLINE OF ITS INTERNAL EXTENSIONS

URETHRAL OPENING

LABIA MINORA

LABIA MAJORA

VAGINAL OPENING

OPENING AND OUTLINE OF BARTHOLIN'S GLAND

REMAINS OF HYMEN

PERINEUM

FOURCHETTE

ANUS

The vulva (external genitals) in *a* an infant and *b* an adult woman, with the labia parted

'clean', you may have learnt to find your own musky smell unpleasant when, in fact, it could be surprisingly arousing to a sexual partner. The amount of moisture in this area and the degree to which odour is noticeable will change during the menstrual cycle – of that, more later.

During sexual excitement, both labia undergo alterations. A

woman who has not given birth will find her labia majora will flatten against her body and almost disappear just before orgasm, while one who has had a baby will find the lips swelling to as much as two to three times their normal size. The inner lips flush a rich colour in the early stages of excitement – pink in one who has not yet had a pregnancy, and red in one who has. The labia minora will swell to two or three times their normal size, whether or not the woman has given birth.

After menopause, the hair covering the labia majora may become sparser and indeed can follow hair on the head in turning grey. Both labia are likely to lose some of their tissue and become thinner. The amount of moisture exuded will probably decline and the skin covering the labia may become friable and less elastic.

## THE CLITORIS

To the front of the vulva, the labia minora come together to form a protective hood around the clitoris. This organ corresponds to the male penis in many ways in that it is the primary site of sexual pleasure. Like the penis, it becomes erect and particularly sensitive during sexual excitement. The clitoris is present and responsive in a pre-pubertal girl, but around half the size it will be in the mature state. There is a belief that women are capable of experiencing greater pleasure in sexual intercourse than men and the structure of the clitoris could support this. The word clitoris derives from the Greek 'to hide' or 'to enclose', and packed into its 4–5 mm. there is a net of sensitive nerve endings three times as large as that of the penis in proportion to its size. The average penis enlarges by around 50 per cent during sexual stimulation. Although some women experience engorgement without an increase in size, the average clitoris enlarges by as much as two- to three-fold. Furthermore, a thin but lengthy band of erectile tissue passes from the clitoris itself backwards and downwards into the body, separating and sweeping round the vagina. Many women derive their sexual satisfaction from stimulation of this area during sexual intercourse rather than direct manipulation of the clitoris. Even women who have experienced the mutilating operation of female circumcision, which removes the clitoris itself, are still capable of some sexual satisfaction from stimulation of this network of nerves.

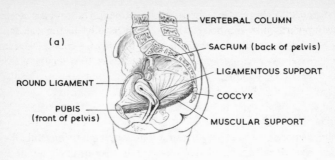

(a)

VERTEBRAL COLUMN

SACRUM (back of pelvis)

LIGAMENTOUS SUPPORT

ROUND LIGAMENT

COCCYX

PUBIS
(front of pelvis)

MUSCULAR SUPPORT

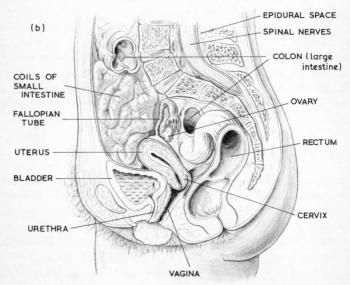

(b)

EPIDURAL SPACE

SPINAL NERVES

COLON (large
intestine)

COILS OF
SMALL
INTESTINE

OVARY

FALLOPIAN
TUBE

UTERUS

RECTUM

BLADDER

URETHRA

CERVIX

VAGINA

The female reproductive organs, showing *a* the protective boney surrounds of
the pelvis, and the supporting ligaments, and *b* the organs that surround the
uterus, seen from the side

## THE URETHRA

Behind the clitoris is the urethra or water passage from which the
body's waste water is expelled. The urethra is usually hidden by the
labia which touch each other when a woman has her legs together.

The opening to the urethra forms a narrow slit. The urethra itself passes upwards into the body, at first lying parallel to the vagina. This narrow, muscular tube lined with a mucous coat is about 3.7 cm. long. Its upper part curves slightly forward to enter the bladder.

## THE BLADDER

The bladder is the reservoir for our waste water or urine and is a flexible, elastic sac capable of holding up to three-quarters of a pint of liquid. It lies in the pelvic cavity in front of and slightly below the uterus. Its lower back wall lies next to the top half of the vagina and the cervix. In infancy, the bladder is the shape of a cone. The adult bladder, when empty, would be cup-shaped and when slightly expanded rounds out, becoming oval when full. Moderately distended it would measure about 12–13 cm. long and 7–8 cm. across. When it does fill up, it is the front wall that curves outwards, which is why you can feel a full bladder almost pushing against your lower belly. The bladder is made of layers of muscular fibre and is lined with a thin, smooth, pale pink mucous coat. Its outer layer is thick and rubbery.

## THE VAGINAL OPENING

Behind the opening to the urethra, also concealed unless the labia are parted, is the opening of the vagina. In a woman who has not had sexual penetration, this opening is often partially blocked by a thin membrane – the hymen or maidenhead. This membrane varies considerably from woman to woman. In some, it forms a fairly tough obstruction and in unusual cases even totally blocks the opening. This is called an imperforate hymen. Sometimes it is laced across the vagina, making several openings. In other women, the hymen is hardly noticeable at all or has been stretched or broken by exploration or masturbation.

Also just inside the vagina are the two Bartholin's Glands which lie under the surface one either side of the entrance. They cannot usually be seen or felt and would only be apparent if swollen by infection or a cyst. In the same way as the ovaries are the female version of the testicles, and the clitoris analogous to the male penis, so the Bartholin's Glands mirror a man's Cowper Glands, which produce a clear fluid during sexual excitement to make intercourse easy and pleasant. The Bartholin's Glands react to stimulation by passing lubrication into the lower end of the vagina via two narrow ducts. This fluid also seeps out to add to the moisture from the sebaceous and apocrine glands, making the labia shiny and flexible.

## THE RECTUM

Behind the vagina, the labia come together to form the fourchette, a ridge of soft tissue, which disappears after childbirth. The perineum – a smooth, flat area – lies between this and the anus (the opening to the rectum or solid-waste passage). The rectum is the final part of the alimentary canal or gastro-intestinal tract, an 11-metre long tube that stretches from your mouth to your anus. On its route through your body this tube widens out to become the stomach and colon and narrows to become the small and large intestine. The majority of its length is compressed in twisting coils inside your abdomen, filling the space not occupied by other organs and virtually surrounding the internal female reproductive organs. The rectum itself is around 20 cm. long and when empty is held flat by the pressure of the surrounding organs. The rectum is capable of being stretched quite considerably. It consists of four coats; a thick rubbery outer coat, muscular fibre, mucous and muscular layers and, finally, mucous membrane. This lining falls into folds when the rectum is empty and so not stretched. Waste matter is forced down through the small and large intestine by a process called peristalsis. The muscles in the walls of the digestive tube contract and relax in a rhythmic, wave-like motion forcing matter along. This movement is not under your conscious control. However, when waste reaches the rectum, you do have some say. There is a ring of muscle surrounding the anus or opening to the rectum, called the anal sphincter. Although in newborn babies and infants the relaxing of this muscle is an automatic reaction to a full rectum, in adults the sphincter normally only responds to conscious effort. Peristalsis may fill the rectum but, in most cases, you empty it by directing your sphincter to open and by contracting the muscles in your diaphragm or upper belly to force a motion out. The food you eat and the lifestyle you lead can have a dramatic effect on your bowel movements. A high-fibre diet will lead to bulkier and easier movements.

## THE VAGINA

The vagina is a flexible tube reaching some 10 cm. into the woman's body. When standing, the vagina would extend upwards and backwards along a line drawn from the vulva towards the small of the back. The word derives from the Latin for 'sheath', an interesting definition since it shows what the original labellers saw as its *chief* function: a scabbard for the 'sword' or male organ! The lower wall of the vagina is known as the posterior wall and is usually about 7 to 10 cm. long. Most women would be able to reach to the vaginal vault which is the end of the tube. The front or anterior wall is shorter, at around 6 to 8 cm., being interrupted by the cervix or neck of the womb that juts out into the vagina at this point.

The vagina is lined with a special covering of cells called squamous epithelium. These are thin and scaly, unlike the thicker and smoother skin on the outside of our bodies. When all is well, they have a pink and shiny appearance. The cells form a mucous membrane, moistened constantly by a fluid that oozes through the walls and keeps it flexible. This white, opaque fluid is acidic and consists of glycogen (a form of sugar), discarded cells from the top layer of tissue and a type of helpful organism called Doederlein's bacilli. These convert the glycogen to lactic acid, which inhibits the growth of many infections. This extraordinary self-cleansing mechanism makes douching or washing out the vagina a very bad idea: it is unnecessary and is more likely to clean away helpful fluid than anything else.

Vaginal secretion changes in amount and appearance during the menstrual cycle and over a woman's lifetime. It often seeps from the vagina to leave a white or cream stain on underclothes. Before puberty, the vagina does not produce a discharge. The first appearance of one is often an early sign that menarche or the first period is approaching. At this stage it is likely to be particularly opaque and is thus often referred to as 'The Whites'. This form may persist for about two years, until ovulation has been established and vaginal fluid is affected by the further addition of mucus from the cervix, as described later in this chapter.

Vaginal lubrication will increase at times, such as during sexual excitement or under the stimulus of physical exertion or nervousness. There may also be an increase during menstruation or as a pregnancy progresses. Just before a period, the vaginal secretion can take on a fine, creamy, granular appearance, somewhat like semolina pudding.

This is caused by increase in the shedding of epithelial cells. Vaginal secretions normally have a fairly noticeable smell that is not unpleasant. When fresh, the odour is slightly musky or can remind you of the seashore. When you have been unable to wash this area for some time, it can become 'fishy'. Far from showing a lack of hygiene or being offensive, the fresh smell is actually attractive and sexually exciting to the opposite sex. After menopause, the secretion may lessen and the walls of the vagina can become thinner, paler in colour, less flexible and quite fragile.

The vagina is at its narrowest in the first few centimetres of its length. Towards the upper two-thirds it widens and during sexual excitement will even 'balloon out'. The lower third is rich in nerve endings, while the area towards the top and around the cervix is far less sensitive. These are the reasons you will feel a tampon as you insert it but may not be aware of its presence once it is in place high in the vagina – and, incidentally, why penis size is largely irrelevant.

## THE CERVIX

Jutting out into the vagina through its anterior or upper wall is the cervix. This is the neck or end of the womb or uterus. The uterus itself is a pear-shaped, pear-sized bag which lies stem-end down in your pelvic cavity, the stem being the cervix. The cervix itself lies around 6 to 8 cm. inside your body and is about 2.5 cm. long. In a woman who has not had a pregnancy, the cervix will be round and cone-shaped, with a tiny circular hole down the middle. This is the os or cervical canal – the opening to the uterus. After birth, or if a late abortion has taken place, the os will resemble a mouth-like slit with an upper and lower lip, and the cervix will become oval-shaped and larger than before. The cervix produces its own mucus, a clear, colourless, alkaline secretion that blocks up the os. This acts as a barrier against infection and against sperm. The cervix is normally firm to touch and the os is tightly closed. An object such as a finger, a tampon or a penis could not possibly pass through this narrow channel.

As ovulation approaches, at about the midway point between your periods, the cervix will soften and produce a greater amount of mucus. This can be of such a quantity that it is known as the 'ovulatory cascade'. Most women will be able to notice that around this time their vaginal discharge becomes thinner and more slippery in texture.

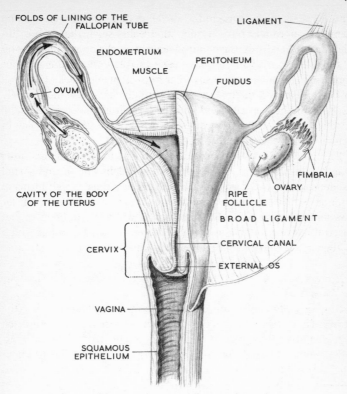

FOLDS OF LINING OF THE
FALLOPIAN TUBE

LIGAMENT

ENDOMETRIUM

MUSCLE

PERITONEUM

FUNDUS

OVUM

CAVITY OF THE BODY
OF THE UTERUS

RIPE
FOLLICLE

FIMBRIA

OVARY

BROAD LIGAMENT

CERVIX

CERVICAL CANAL

EXTERNAL OS

VAGINA

SQUAMOUS
EPITHELIUM

Back view of the uterus, vagina, fallopian tubes and ovaries

This is a result of the increased flow of cervical mucus combining with vaginal secretions. Instead of plugging the os, this mucus forms channels to speed sperm on its way and becomes far more acidic, giving maximum opportunity for sperm survival. Cervical secretion contains proteins and sugars which actually sustain sperm on its journey. The cervix will also secrete more fluid under the impetus of sexual excitement and, along with the Bartholin's Glands, may go on pouring out moisture up to twenty-four hours after arousal.

The surface of the cervix is similar to that of the vagina – covered in squamous epithelium. The os, however, is lined with glandular mucous membrane. This is only a single layer in thickness and the cells are larger and more active than the tissue lining the vagina and the cervix. They look far rougher and are coloured a deeper red. After a pregnancy or being on the Pill, the cervix may become darker in colour and some of the cells lining the os may move outwards on to the surface of the cervix, giving it a more grainy appearance. After menopause, the cervix follows the changes in the vagina and will become paler in colour.

## THE UTERUS

The uterus itself is about 5 cm. long – 7.5 cm. including the cervix – in a woman who has not yet had a pregnancy. Its walls are around 1.2 cm. thick and the cavity, which is normally compressed shut, is about 3.7 cm. long. Obviously, the uterus is immensely flexible: if this cavity is filled by a developing baby and its protective surroundings, it expands. After birth, it remains slightly bigger than before the event.

Before puberty, the pear-shaped organ is about half its adult size and it grows as part of the changes that occur during adolescence. The uterus hangs in the centre of the pelvic cavity and is normally pitched forward, with the cervix pointing backwards and downwards towards the buttocks. When you stand upright and your bladder is empty, the uterus will be lying almost horizontal inside you. It does not float around in empty space but is cushioned on all sides by the other organs in this area. Below the front wall lies the bladder, while above and around are the coils of the bowel, the rectum or back passage and the vagina.

The uterus is held in place by the projection of the cervix into the vagina and by ligaments or bands of strong tissue. These are slung across the pelvic cavity from the pelvic walls, the rectum and the bladder. They support and secure the uterus, fallopian tubes and the ovaries. However, the uterus is not fixed rigidly in place and does move around a surprising amount. When the bladder is full, the uterus will be pushed backwards, and a full rectum will push it down and forwards again. Depending on whether you are standing or lying, your uterus will settle under the force of gravity. During sexual excitement, the ligaments tighten to lift it out of the way of a thrusting penis. Even breathing will pull the uterus up and down in time with respiratory movement.

The uterus is covered in a thick, rubbery coat called the peritoneum. Underneath this is a layer of muscle marbled with lymphatic and blood vessels and nerves. This runs in a band up the front of the uterus, over the top and back down to the cervix. It is not under conscious control, but flexes and contracts in response to chemical messages during orgasm, labour or menstruation. Scattered through-out the tissue in the walls of the uterus are smaller muscles. Their function is to periodically shut off small blood vessels leading to the inner lining of the womb, leaving it to decay and come away each month as the menstrual flow. At the end of a period these muscles contract further, to stop the bleeding.

The entire uterine cavity is lined with endometrial tissue, which is soft, pink and rich in blood vessels. During each menstrual cycle, the endometrium thickens and grows until menstruation, when it comes away as the menstrual flow. The amount of fluid lost can be from 50 to 175 cc – around a quarter to three-quarters of a cup. The flow consists of blood, degenerated cells and mucus. The uterine cavity does not 'store up' blood. If the period is a little heavier than usual, that will be because the endometrial lining has become thicker, not because blood has been blocked or held back inside you. Similarly, a light period – such as many women experience while on the Pill, for example – is a result of the lining having been thinner in that month.

The uterus not only changes its position depending on the physical attitude of the woman and the state of the surrounding organs, but its appearance and texture change in response to the menstrual cycle and to the woman's age. It will be larger and rounder during a period and will become firmer and bulkier in the early stages of pregnancy. After menopause, it shrinks slightly and becomes paler in colour.

## THE FALLOPIAN TUBES

The uterus becomes progessively wider from the cervix to the fundus or top. Here, it opens out on either side into the fallopian tubes. These extend for some 10 to 16 cm. out from the uterus, curving round to partly encircle the ovaries. The fallopian tubes end in finger-like projections called fimbria. These hover over the ovaries, coming closer as ovulation approaches. The fallopian tubes are attached to liga-ments that also anchor the uterus. The tube is a narrow, muscular channel, lined with mucous membrane. Some of the cells composing this lining are 'ciliated' – that is, they seem almost hair-like. The cilia move and wave, like the arms of a sea anemone. This sets up a current in the fluids circulating in the pelvic cavity, from the ovary down the fallopian tubes and into the uterus.

## THE OVARIES

Hanging from the ligaments near the open ends of the fallopian tubes are the ovaries. These are approximately the size and shape of almonds, around 3.5 cm. long and 2 cm. wide. Before puberty, they are shiny and smooth in appearance and become progressively roughened and puckered during the reproductive years. They are a bluish-white colour and shrink and harden after menopause. At birth, each ovary will contain around 100,000 follicles – the immature cells that could develop into an ovum or egg and combine with male sperm to become a baby. At puberty, around 30,000 follicles remain, of which some 400 might develop fully during a woman's reproductive lifetime.

From puberty, each month, several follicles start to mature. The trigger for this development is the release into the bloodstream of various hormones – the chemical messengers produced by glands in our bodies. The development of the female body from child to woman, and the day-to-day progress of the menstrual cycle, are controlled primarily by two glands at the base of the brain – the hypothalamus and the pituitary. These provide – among other things – the stimulus for the immature body to gain weight and for the mature body to ovulate, menstruate, go into labour and produce milk from the breasts.

We are still not entirely certain what it is that triggers puberty and the beginning of periods – the menarche. There appears to be some link with the proportion of body fat to weight, but the relationship and the mechanism are by no means clear. You are likely to find, however, that you follow your mother's pattern and that any daughters of yours will have a similar menstrual history. Women who have an early menarche are also likely to have a late menopause.

## THE HYPOTHALAMUS
## AND THE PITUITARY

The relationship of the hypothalamus and pituitary to the reproductive system is complex and extremely sensitive. The hypothalamus functions as a regulator, producing releasing agents to prompt the pituitary to manufacture hormones of its own and to stimulate further production elsewhere in the body. In turn, the hypothalamus is responsive to the physical and emotional state of

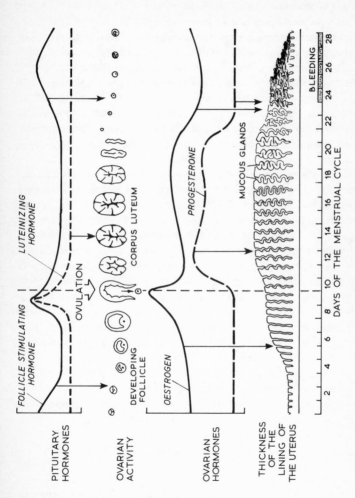

Hormone levels and their effects during the menstrual cycle when pregnancy does not take place

the body as a whole. Women who are under stress, in poor health or suffering a drastic loss or gain in weight are likely to find their entire hormonal system affected.

From puberty, each month, the pituitary will start the menstrual cycle by producing a hormone called follicle stimulating hormone (FSH). Several follicles will begin to ripen in the ovaries. As these grow, they secrete a second hormone, oestrogen. This acts on the lining of the uterus, causing it to thicken and grow. Oestrogen can also make the breasts and vagina sensitive. After six to eight days, the pituitary stops producing FSH and starts secreting luteinizing hormone (LH). This stimulates one of the follicles to burst open on the surface of the ovary and to release an ovum or egg. This is ovulation. Usually, only one follicle will mature, but sometimes two sites rupture at the same time, producing two ova. If these are fertilized and come to term, the result would be non-identical twins. One in 87 pregnancies is of twins, three-quarters of them being formed in this way. The other 25 per cent are identical twins, created by the splitting in two of one fertilized ovum.

The ovum will be caught in the circulating fluid and wafted towards and down the fallopian tube. If the egg is to be fertilized, it needs to meet living, vigorous sperm near the end of the fallopian tube. Since sperm travel at about 2.5 cm. per hour, this would mean that conception itself can occur some ten to twelve hours after intercourse. The egg takes time to travel down the fallopian tube to the uterus – around seven to eight days – and has a 'shelf life' of around twelve to twenty-four hours. Sperm lives for up to three days, so providing intercourse takes place some time between three days before or a day after ovulation, conception is a possibility.

After the ovum has burst out of the ovary, the follicle it has left becomes the 'corpus luteum', the production site for yet another hormone – progesterone. This hormone primes the sites already prepared for a pregnancy and prevents the further maturation and release of more eggs. If the egg is fertilized, it in turn secretes a hormone into the woman's bloodstream. This is called human chorionic gonadatrophin (HCG), and it sustains the corpus luteum and encourages the continued production of progesterone and so maintains the pregnancy. We can detect pregnancy at a very early stage now by looking for minute quantities of HCG excreted in urine.

If the egg is not fertilized, the corpus luteum breaks up after seven days and ceases to produce progesterone. Some fourteen days after

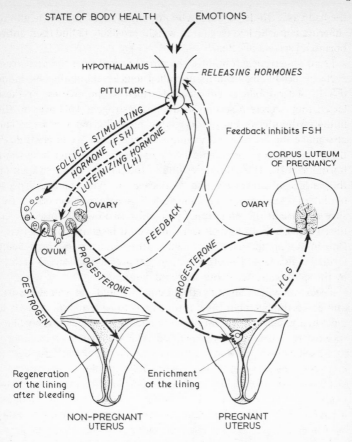

STATE OF BODY HEALTH    EMOTIONS

HYPOTHALAMUS —

— *RELEASING HORMONES*

PITUITARY

*FOLLICLE STIMULATING HORMONE (FSH)*

*LUTEINIZING HORMONE (LH)*

Feedback inhibits FSH

CORPUS LUTEUM OF PREGNANCY

OVARY

OVARY

*FEEDBACK*

*PROGESTERONE*

*PROGESTERONE*

*H.C.G.*

OVUM

*OESTROGEN*

Regeneration of the lining after bleeding

Enrichment of the lining

NON-PREGNANT UTERUS

PREGNANT UTERUS

All the hormones are bloodborne and partially excreted in the urine, where they can be detected

The interaction of the female hormones on the non-pregnant and early pregnant uterus

ovulation, the muscles in the sides of the uterus respond to the drop in progesterone levels by closing up and cutting off supply to the endometrium. This then comes away as a flow of blood, tissue and fluid as FSH levels begin to pick up, starting the whole cycle over again.

The menstrual cycle is often a good guide to a woman's well-being. Periods may be irregular during adolescence but usually settle into some sort of rhythm in the late teens. For convenience we tend to talk about the menstrual cycle as lasting twenty-eight days, and the Combined Oral Contraceptive Pill imposes a four-week cycle by giving you twenty-one days of pill-taking followed by seven pill-free days during which a bleed occurs. In fact, the normal range – from the first day of bleeding to the last day before the next bleed – can be from twenty-one to thirty-five days, with an average spread of twenty-five to thirty days.

## ——— *BREASTS* ———

Breasts are called 'secondary sexual characteristics', since they are not central to the primary role of our sexual organs which is to produce young. However, this label underestimates the importance most of us place on this part of our body, for breasts are not only sources of nourishment for a baby, but are also a focus for sexual attractiveness. In both these functions, breasts can be seen as having enormous significance. A woman who has small breasts or who has difficulty – or thinks she may be having difficulty – in breastfeeding, is quite likely to feel that her femininity is in question.

Breasts are probably more on public display now in the Western world than at any time in our recorded history. Not only are 'topless' beaches accepted in most tourist resorts, but the Western media show the naked breast in advertisements, films and television programmes as a matter of course. Sadly, instead of showing the diversity of breast size and shape, this has led many people to expect a 'normal' breast to conform to a standard. Rather like the supermarket apple, we all expect to see a 'Eurobreast'! Media breasts tend to be medium sized, firm, hairless, uniformly coloured and with erect, pink nipples. What the consumer cannot see are the tricks of the trade that produce this image. Invisible tape can be employed to ensure the breast does not droop and that the nipples point upwards, and the nipples themselves are persuaded to stand firm by the application of an ice cube or a spray of water. Stretchmarks and veins are covered by make-up or air-brushed out of the finished photograph.

In fact, breasts come in all shapes and sizes, from the firm apples, pears or plums to the soft beanbags. Nipples and the surrounding areola range from a delicate pink to a dark brown – the colour changing and darkening either temporarily with stimulus or permanently with pregnancy and age. Nipples themselves are made of erectile tissue that fills with blood and becomes firm and stands out under stimulus. The stimulus can be sexual excitement, nervousness or fear, physical exertion, cold or just the sensation of being touched or rubbed, for instance by loose clothing. When not stimulated, the nipple is soft and flat or even dimpled.

Until puberty, the breast area of both boys and girls has a similar appearance – flat chest with small, pink nipples ringed by rose-hued, nubbled skin. Both sexes can even have extra nipples, occurring anywhere on the line from the armpit, down the chest under the breasts. In medieval days these were thought to be the sign of a witch (male or female) who would suckle demons from them.

The breast itself is made up of fat, tissue and milk ducts. During puberty, as the female body responds to hormonal changes, layers of fat will accumulate on hips, thighs and the chest area. The areola – the area of soft skin surrounding the nipple – will begin to bulge as milk ducts and pads of fat grow inwards underneath the skin, pushing the breast outwards from the chest wall. After around eighteen months, the breast is fully formed in its adult shape and size.

The areola changes from pink to dark brown or even black around the second month of a first pregnancy and, although the colour will lighten after the birth, will remain darker afterwards. The areola is dotted with 'goose pimples' which are actually sebaceous glands – oil-producing glands which secrete a fatty substance to keep the area flexible and lubricated. This is especially important during breastfeeding and at this time the glands become more active and prominent and are known as Montgomery's Tubercles.

A ring of fine hair surrounds the nipple, hair that will be light and almost invisible in some women; dark, coarse and obvious in others. During puberty, the pale, downy fuzz that covers all our bodies will thicken and coarsen under arms, in the pubic area, and on the limbs of adults of both sexes. Depending on your particular colouring and racial type, women as well as men may find dark hair growing on their chests and this is neither abnormal nor a sign that they are in any way masculinized.

The nipple is made up of tissues and fibres which will engorge with blood when stimulated. The surface of the nipple is pierced with tiny openings which lead to the milk reservoirs. The breast contains milk-producing cells called alveoli which cluster together in lobules. The lobules themselves gather in fifteen to twenty lobes, held together by fibrous tissue and separated from each other by pads of fat. Lactiferous

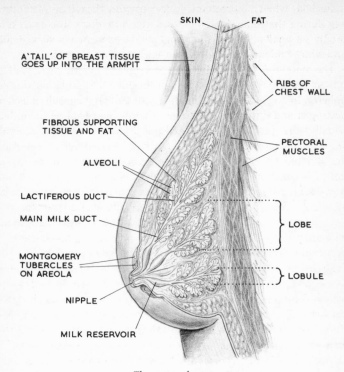

SKIN

FAT

A'TAIL' OF BREAST TISSUE
GOES UP INTO THE ARMPIT

RIBS OF
CHEST WALL

FIBROUS SUPPORTING
TISSUE AND FAT

PECTORAL
MUSCLES

ALVEOLI

LACTIFEROUS DUCT

MAIN MILK DUCT

LOBE

MONTGOMERY
TUBERCLES
ON AREOLA

LOBULE

NIPPLE

MILK RESERVOIR

The mature breast

ducts carry the milk from lobules into one of the main ducts leading from each lobe to a nipple, and these widen just before the nipple to form milk reservoirs.

Breasts contain no muscle at all, which is why no amount of exercise or therapy will increase their size. There is a sheet of muscle – the pectoral muscle – which lies between the breast and the chest wall. This can indeed be firmed and enlarged by exercise, providing a firmer platform from which the breasts can hang, but having no effect on breast size itself. The shape and size of your breasts is largely determined by the amount of fatty tissue you have, enlarging or decreasing in size as you gain or lose weight. Pregnancy and breastfeeding, of course, will often increase their size as the milk ducts come into action. These ducts are often also stimulated by the oral contraceptive pill. The Combined Pill works by mimicking the hormone levels present in the body when it is pregnant, so discouraging the release of another egg during that time. In some cases, the milk ducts also react and produce a small amount of milk that can be expressed or sucked out, and which can make the breasts appear larger and firmer.

The amount of milk-producing and supportive tissue each woman has in her breasts is determined by hormonal stimulation during puberty. In a very few cases, small breasts can be the result of lack of oestrogen and if this is so oestrogen therapy can enlarge them, but usually only if treatment is carried out before maturity. In general, size and shape is related to overall body build. Most developing women find that one breast outstrips its companion by as much as a cup size and it is common even after full growth is completed to have one breast larger than the other and for their shape and texture not to be identical. Breasts alter in size, shape and appearance throughout a woman's lifetime, and during the menstrual cycle, and changes can be permanent or temporary. The most noticeable permanent effects occur under the influnce of age, menopause and pregnancy.

During pregnancy, blood-supply to the breasts increases by around 20 per cent. Not only does the milk-producing tissue grow and fill up, but the fat stores increase in order to nourish the mother as she feeds her baby. By the time the baby is born, breasts may be as much as a third larger than normal. The size of the breast is no indication of the amount of milk available, since much of the bulk is cushioning fat rather than milk ducts. Small breasts can give as much milk as large ones. After the baby is weaned, the milk ducts will shrink and stop working and the breasts will return to their former size, the extra fat having been converted to energy. The remaining tissue may feel softer and the breast be slacker. Faint silvery lines called stria will mark the increase and decrease in size. The marks are caused by minute bundles of fibres *under* the skin having been stretched and broken, so no amount of creams, oils or lotions massaged into the surface will have any effect on their appearance.

As women age, the fibrous breast tissues slacken. After menopause, the milk-producing and -carrying ducts shrink, and the whole breast can become smaller and softer. In some cases, fat replaces these tissues so overall size is not lost but firmness will almost certainly lessen and the texture of both breast and skin will change.

Pregnancy causes both temporary and permanent changes to breasts, but an even more startling but short-lived change is produced by sexual excitement. When a woman is sexually stimulated, the nipples become erect and the areola appear to enlarge and flush a dark colour. Indeed, the whole chest area can become mottled and the veins become dramatically visible. Just before orgasm, the breast itself can swell by as much as a quarter, especially in women who have not yet breastfed. This effect is often exploited by companies offering breast enlarging methods. Massaging the area with cream or cold water sprays *will* have a sufficiently stimulating effect to mimic sexual excitement and if this arousal is not satisfied, the condition can be maintained for some hours. However, it soon returns to normal and sexual excitement itself never causes any lasting changes to the body.

The size and texture of your breasts are also likely to change during your menstrual cycle. Just before your period, the milk ducts can respond to hormonal changes by thickening and becoming lumpy or rubbery. Breasts may also feel tender and be slightly larger at this time. We will be looking further at the implications of these changes in Chapter 3.

This chapter should have given you a rough idea of what to expect when looking at your body and an understanding of how it works when all is well. In the next chapter we shall be considering some of the things that can go wrong.

──────── CHAPTER 2 ────────

# What Can Go Wrong

T he female body does appear to be depressingly vulnerable to disease, infection and irritating disorders. However, women are by at least one parameter 'healthier' than men in having a life expectancy of an extra six years. Just because in this book we are examining the problems that *can* affect the female body – and specifically the female sexual and reproductive organs – do not jump to the conclusion that women are inherently disease-prone or are necessarily weak.

Unlike the male body, the female body does change regularly. One of our difficulties is in taking ourselves seriously and in sorting out the changes that are symptoms of a problem from those that are a part of a woman's normal cycle. Any confusion is not helped by the fact that the medical profession was hijacked several centuries ago by men. Medical definitions and attitudes unconsciously take the male body as the norm. Look up a diagram in a medical textbook illustrating any part of the body that is common to both sexes, and the body pictured will *always* be male! The female body is only used when it is specifically female organs that are being shown.

So to be well and normal is to be stable and unchanging. The Old Wise Women knew that women altered with the moon and that such fluctuations should be accepted and even celebrated, but traditional medicine disagrees. In effect, a woman is an 'ill man'. The changes in our bodies periodically attract our attention, but instead of embracing this and using it as a way of becoming more aware of ourselves, we call such reminders 'the curse'. We allow men to dismiss the ebb and flow of our physical and emotional state as neurotic or hysterical, but above all abnormal. Discussion of a perfectly normal event which happens to 52 per cent of the world's population thirteen times a year is taboo, and we largely remain too embarrassed to seek information. The result is that many of us flounder in a confused state, frightened that some perfectly normal aspect might be the symptom of disease, or too shy to ask for help with the genuine precursor of an illness.

We need to learn which changes are normal, which are similar to expected alterations but need some attention, and which are signals for action. We need to know which symptoms can be dealt with by our own direct or indirect self-help measures, and which need medical intervention. We also need the confidence to ask for health screening when it is appropriate, since some disease is asymptomatic – showing no obvious outward signs – and can only be picked up with professional tests. Many of the problems that affect our reproductive organs have similar symptoms, and some have symptoms that are masked by the ordinary day-to-day or year-to-year changes. We need to feel confident in understanding which of the degenerative changes that occur during the menopause are part of life's rich tapestry, and which we should refuse to put up with at any price! Above all, we need the reassurance that becoming aware of a problem and seeking help for it is *worthwhile*. Even the most extreme conditions, such as cancer, *can* be cured and are not necessarily killers. But illness has to be detected and treated *early* to be controlled, and many infections that start off as a minor condition – such as cystitis – can become progressively more serious if left alone.

At the end of this chapter, we will list the more obvious conditions and give their symptoms and their probable causes. Here, we will follow the previous chapter in progressing through the genitals, from vulva to ovaries and on to the breasts, looking at the symptoms you may notice and discussing what they could mean.

## THE VULVA

The labia minora and the inside of the labia majora are moist and sticky with the oil produced by the sebaceous glands that are rich in this area. After menopause, when the fatty tissue atrophies and decreases, these glands may also dry up and the surface area become paler in colour and dry in texture. The area may then be more delicate and prone to bruising and infection. Before the menopause, dryness in the vulva can accompany vaginal dryness and discomfort. Various infections can trigger redness, soreness and itching and the appearance of open sores in the vulva. An itching and rash when accompanied by a general feeling of being unwell but with no vaginal discharge might indicate an infestation of pubic lice or crabs. These are usually passed on from sexual partners in intimate contact, although it is possible to catch them from close but non-sexual contact, and from the bedding or clothing of an infested person. Pubic lice are very small but are visible to the naked eye and their eggs are found glued to the shaft of pubic hair. Lice are fairly easily treated. Shampoos or lotions such as Quellada or Prioderm can be bought over the counter in a chemist, and if used according to the instructions they will clear up the attack. Never try a 'do-it-yourself' measure such as putting disinfectants in the bath water. This will not rid you of the lice, but will almost certainly upset the delicate balance of organisms on the vulva and in the vagina, worsening or leading to infection. If the vagina is also affected by the rash and irritation, thrush or trichomoniasis is more likely – of these, more later.

Just as sebaceous glands on the face can become blocked and infected, so too can those on the vulva. This may result in a sore, red spot with an infected, pus-filled head – exactly like acne or spots on the face. An open sore, however, may be more sinister. An ulcer that fails to heal or an irregular lump may even be vulval cancer. A hard, painless lesion could be a chancre – the first symptom of syphilis. Itchy, burning or tingling sensations in the vulva that resolve into a single pinprick sore or a cluster of them might indicate herpes. Herpes sores or vesicles often develop acne-like heads filled with a clear liquid, which may burst and scab over. In both syphilis and herpes, the vulva may become swollen, and with herpes this is accompanied by tenderness and sometimes fever.

Another, often painless, external symptom may be genital warts – small bundles of cells growing on the labia and around the anus. They can also occur inside the vagina and on the cervix. Warts are becoming more common – some 40 per cent of women have the human papillomavirus which causes them. The virus may be passed by intimate genital contact or by hand. They can be troublesome in that they may be torn or knocked during sexual activity, bleed painfully and become inflamed or obvious sites for further infections. More worrying, there appears to be a link between having genital warts and developing cancer of the cervix. It has been found that one in thirty women infected by human papillomavirus develop tumours. For this reason, they should not be ignored.

## THE URETHRA AND BLADDER

Pain on passing water is a fairly common complaint and can be the result of damage or infection in the urethra or the bladder. More usually, it is both together since the urethra is so short that any infection in this tube often climbs into the bladder and, if neglected, may continue on into the kidneys. Urethritis or inflammation of the urethra can arise in several situations. The delicate lining can be bruised and torn during sexual intercourse. If love-making is rough or inexpert or the woman's vagina is dry, both the walls of the vagina and the adjacent urethra can be damaged. This is often known as 'honeymoon' cystitis since it frequently happens when a couple are new to sex or new to each other.

Urethritis can also arise from infection by harmful organisms. You can infect yourself by introducing undesirable material into the urethra by wiping yourself from your anus forwards across your vulva after a bowel movement. Bacteria such as E.coli, which thrive harmlessly in the back passage, are likely to inflame both the urethra and the vagina if brought forwards in this way. A sexual partner can inadvertently pass such material to you, or carry your own bacteria on hands, mouth or genitals from one part of your body to another. Using the diaphragm as your method of contraception can also increase your risks of having cystitis, as the hard rim of the device can press against the bladder and urethra through the thin walls of the vagina, causing irritation and inflammation.

If the infection climbs into the bladder, it is known as cystitis. Cystitis is extremely common. As many as one in two women suffer from it at some time. As well as pain on passing water, this can lead to your urine having a cloudy, dark or even bloodstained appearance and to your having a constant urge to urinate, even when you have nothing to pass.

Cystitis and urethritis can also be a response to a sexually transmitted disease, and trichomoniasis and gonorrhoea can both lead to painful urination. Frequently, however, the precise virus or bacteria responsible for an attack of cystitis or urethritis becomes difficult to pin down and in these cases the cause is called N S U (non-specific urethritis). It is now believed that in many of these cases the culprit may be the chlamydia organism which will be discussed later. 'Itis' means inflammation; urethritis, cystitis or vaginitis are terms that simply state you have an inflammation in that particular part of the body.

## THE VAGINA AND CERVIX

Another fairly common symptom is pain in the vagina. Sometimes vaginal pain is only obvious during a physical examination or when the woman attempts to have intercourse. In a woman or girl who has not had previous sexual intercourse, this can arise because the thin membrane partially obstructing the vaginal opening resists. If this has not been stretched by masturbation or the use of tampons or has flexed only to some extent, it may tear painfully when intercourse is attempted for the first time and continue to be tender over several further attempts. While some women may find the hymen stretches, others may find it breaks and bleeds. Vaginal pain can also be a symptom of infection, whether sexually transmitted or otherwise. Frequently, you can learn more about the source of infection by seeing whether pain is accompanied by an unusual vaginal discharge. After the menopause, intercourse can become painful as the vaginal tissues become drier and more delicate. Of both of these, more later.

Painful intercourse can also be attributed to emotional difficulties. Vaginismus is a situation in which the muscles surrounding the vaginal opening and in the vaginal walls clamp shut when approached by an intruding finger, speculum, tampon or penis. Although these muscles are usually under your conscious control, in vaginismus the reaction is involuntary. It is usually a result of hidden fears or painful memories and often needs sympathetic help from a counsellor and the sexual partner, and a commitment on the part of the sufferer to come to terms with what is happening.

Childbirth can also make the vagina sore for some time after the event. The tissue can be bruised and stretched, making it tender, and if stitches were required for an episiotomy or cut, or a tear made in the perineum – the area behind the vaginal opening – this scar tissue can be sore for a considerable period. It can take scar tissue up to eighteen months to mature and settle down, and for this time the area can be scratchy and painful.

It is unfortunate that many of us are taught, directly or subtly, that the area between our legs is somehow dirty and to be avoided. Agony aunties and doctors are familiar with the letter or the query from the frightened and often tearful young girl who has spent months if not years since her menarche convinced that a perfectly normal vaginal secretion was a symptom of disease or damage; and the woman who has endured painful infection rather than 'wasting the doctor's time'. Getting to know your vulva and vagina, and becoming familiar with the moisture found in this area, is as essential as learning how to clean your teeth.

An important indication of vaginal health is the state of the natural moisture found there. The vagina, like the mouth, is meant to be moist. The walls are fragile and elastic and constantly exude a clear liquid to keep themselves in a healthy state. This lubrication will change during the course of the menstrual cycle, being thinner and more slippery around ovulation. Most women find they produce more moisture at this time, and just before their period begins. On the whole, vaginal moisture also increases during physical exertion and sexual excitement. However, you may find yourself becoming progressively less moist as you age, and after the menopause, a dry vagina can pose problems. Gentle and regular sexual play can usually ensure that the lubrication in this part of your body remains adequate, but many older women find that a little help is necessary. The situation arises because of a lack of oestrogen which, after menopause, is no longer available from the ovaries. Some doctors are happy to prescribe an oestrogen cream which can restore elasticity and lubrication. Otherwise, many women find that by using a vaginal lubricating cream such as K Y Jelly, Senselle or Durex lubricating jelly they can return to making love and give their bodies a chance to restore 'normal service'.

Pre-menopausal women can also find there are times when vaginal lubrication becomes scant. In some cases, this can be a strong signal from your body that sexual involvement is not welcome. Physical ill health and stress can have this effect, as can unacknowledged anger at or distaste for your sexual partner. Medication can also provoke dryness. The oral contraceptive pill can inhibit secretions, as can drugs prescribed by a doctor for hay fever, stress or diarrhoea – the anti-histamines, phenothiagines and anti-cholinogenics. Antibiotics can also provoke a dry and sore vagina, and during menstruation and just after a pregnancy, vaginal lubrication may well be scarce.

Most women suffer temporary dryness at some time. This does not mean, however, that it is a situation that should be accepted or ignored. If you judge that the probable cause is tiredness, stress, illness or just the fact that you are not entirely happy to be making love at that time to that person, the steps you take can be appropriate. Change your diet for a healthier one, your routine for a less stressful one and even your lover for a more exciting one! In all these cases, you can work out the reason for your body behaving in this way and act on your own or with your sexual partner to better the situation. Using a lubricating cream or jelly, however, should not be a permanent solution. If you find that you need this to prevent every act of love being painful and the condition does not improve, it is advisable to seek the advice and help of your doctor.

More frequently, discharges cause problems by their presence rather than their absence. The fact that the consistency, quantity and colour of vaginal discharge alters during the menstrual cycle and over a woman's lifetime can sometimes mask a change that is the symptom of a problem. This is why it is so important to become familiar with your own cycle so that any unusual alteration is noticed. Such changes can result in an infection that affects the vagina, the cervix or even the uterus itself.

A thin, watery discharge that persists beyond the period surrounding ovulation could indicate gonorrhoea, or a cervical erosion. Gonorrhoea is a sexually transmitted disease (STD) that can be passed on via oral, vaginal or anal sex. The bacteria that cause it thrive in a warm, moist environment and die quickly on exposure to air. This means that it cannot be passed on by non-intimate contact or on lavatory seats or eating utensils. However, it is conceivable that it can be caught by sharing towels, flannels or sponges if contact is immediate, and that it can be passed from genital to genital by hand contact. In the majority of cases, women developing gonorrhoea do *not* show symptoms, or the symptoms go unremarked. The cervix is the site most often infected, and this can trigger an increase in cervical mucus.

A cervical erosion sounds far more dramatic than it actually is. An erosion or, as some doctors now prefer to call it, an ectropion, is a

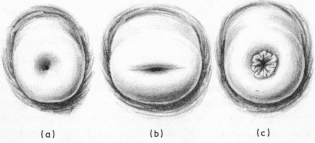

(a)          (b)          (c)

The cervix: *a* before chidbirth; *b* after a pregnancy; *c* with an erosion

reddened area on the surface of the cervix. The cells that line the cervical canal or os are larger and more active than the shiny, pink squamous epithelium that cover the cervix itself. The redder, more roughened mucous membrane is more active and produces greater quantities of lubricating liquid. Frequently, these cells move out of the os on to the surface of the cervix, increasing the area of secretion-producing cells and so the amount of liquid in the vagina. This migration is not the result of damage or disease, which is why the name 'erosion' is so misleading and frightening. It does give the impression that one is being eaten away or has been damaged by over-vigorous intercourse or misuse of a tampon. These changes often happen during puberty, during pregnancy or are just triggered by being on the Pill. In most cases, the erosion resolves itself as the acidic environment of the vagina encourages the area to change into thicker cells. However, erosions are sometimes a nuisance if they persist. The thinner nature of these cells also makes them a target for infection. For this reason, doctors may suggest that erosions be dealt with by cauterization or excision. If the area is cut, burnt or frozen away, it will be replaced by a regrowth of the original, tougher and larger cells.

A thicker, whitish discharge with the appearance of curd cheese is likely to be caused by a thrush infection. Many microscopic organisms inhabit and thrive on the surface and in the cavities of our bodies. When all is well, these live in harmony with us and do not make their presence known. The warm, moist and acid environment of the vagina is home to a yeast-like organism called candida albicans. When the vagina becomes too alkaline, the fungus-like organism can multiply, giving rise to an unpleasant condition called moniliasis or thrush. The vagina and vulva may become itchy and sore; there will probably be patches of the white yeast on the walls of the vagina, and a thick, white, curd-like and yeasty-smelling discharge.

Normal vaginal discharge will also change if there is infection or inflammation in the vagina or on the cervix. Mucous membrane can be damaged and inflamed by douching. Douching used to be con-sidered an effective method of birth-control and an important part of female hygiene. Water, mixed with a proprietary antiseptic or lemon juice, salt or vinegar, or soap, was introduced into the vagina through a rubber bulb or bag fitted with a nozzle or neck. Douching is no longer recommended. Not only is it useless as contraception, it can force harmful bacteria through the os and into the uterus. The vaginal fluids perform their own cleansing, and washing them away leaves the area vulnerable to attack from infection or paves the way for thrush to thrive.

Objects left in the vagina can also irritate the area, and a forgotten diaphragm, cap or tampon can produce problems. If you do experience a foul-smelling discharge, it is always sensible to check first that nothing has been left inside the vagina – at the top where you might not feel its presence. Tampons left too long, or inserted with difficulty into a dry vagina, can in unusual cases lead to a serious infection called toxic shock syndrome (TSS). The bacteria staphylococcus areus can enter into the body through minute wounds caused by the stretching and tearing of tissue, or scratches caused by a tampon inserter tube. Or they can be absorbed through the thin membrane of the vaginal walls, especially if a tampon is left for many hours or has been contaminated by dirty hands before insertion. Symptoms of TSS include sore throat and fever, rash and flushing of the skin, diarrhoea, aching muscles and sore, red eyes.

A bubbly, yellow or green discharge with an unpleasant smell is often the main symptom of another of the bacterial infections that can be sexually transmitted. This is trichomoniasis vaginalis, or 'trich' or 'TV'. It can also make your vagina – and sometimes the vulva and insides of your thighs – red and sore. The discharge can be pale in colour and so mimic that caused by other vaginal infections. Sexually transmitted diseases often travel in pairs or even groups – gonorrhoea is frequently accompanied by trich. Trich can affect the cervix as well as the vagina, as can chlamydia – one of the most elusive and possibly the most troublesome of the cervical infections.

Chlamydia is now thought to be the single, main micro-organism responsible for cases of non-specific genital infections – inflammation for which tests cannot pin down a definite culprit. It was thought that these were primarily a problem for the male partner. We now think that untreated chlamydia results in a large proportion of the cases of PID – pelvic inflammatory disease – which is a major cause of infertility in women and with which we will be dealing later. The first symptom of chlamydia is often slight spotting and a small increase in discharge. The infection may well then become 'silent' until the sufferer has symptoms of PID. The cervix itself may be inflamed, tender and prone to bleeding, and the os blocked with mucus stained with blood. There may be a greyish-white discharge, but this could be masked by the normal flow of lubrication from the vagina.

The cervix is also often the site of infection for Herpes vesicles which, in addition to bursting and weeping, can become further infected and produce an unpleasant discharge. Frequently, however, they can be 'silent', producing no pain and no discharge and so spreading the virus without the infected woman feeling their presence.

Unusual discharges can also be the result of allergies to materials encountered in the vagina, such as those used to make contraceptive sheaths, sponges, diaphragms, caps or spermicides. In some cases, an unusual discharge may indicate the presence of a form of cancer.

## CANCER

The main fear that most people have when finding any unusual or distressing symptom is that it could be cancer. Each cell in your body has a specific task – to be part of the protective skin, or part of the blood-supply or part of a specific organ. Cancer is when cells in your body go 'maverick' and begin to divide and multiply, but to perform no proper function. Cancerous cells are not 'diseased' in the sense of being suppurating or rotten. When they go out of control, they can form a colony of abnormal cells, called a tumour. When a 'malignant' tumour forms, it will spread and cancerous cells will break off from the main mass and migrate through the body's lymphatic system to other areas. These will form new colonies, spreading and growing and taking the place of healthy cells and disrupting their work. This spreading process is called metastasis. Abnormal growths of cells need not be cancerous, however. They may be 'benign' or innocent. A benign tumour has a layer around it and although it may press painfully on surrounding tissue and grow large enough to be a problem, it cannot send colonies of diseased cells to other parts of the body, so its effect is limited.

If you experience discomforting symptoms, cancer should not be your first thought. Cancer of the vagina is quite rare, while cancer of the cervix accounts for only 4 per cent of all cancer deaths. However, the occurrence of changes that could suggest the development of cancer in the cervix – often referred to as pre-malignant changes – seems to have doubled in the last ten years in women in the UK. Cancer of the cervix, like most forms of this disease, is primarily a disease in the older woman. The peak incidence is in the late forties and fifties. This does not mean, however, that younger women never suffer. In the latest figures, around fifty of the 2,000 women in

England and Wales who died from cancer of the cervix in a year were under the age of thirty-six, with six of them under twenty-five. There are suggestions that when younger women do develop cancer, the tumours grow and become malignant more quickly than in older women, but there is as yet no certain confirmation of this theory.

Cancer of the vagina or cervix is asymptomatic in its early stages, but can cause bleeding and a watery, smelly and bloodstained discharge, especially after intercourse. Since older women who have had their menopause are the ones most likely to develop this, a doctor should be seen immediately if you have vaginal bleeding after your periods have ceased, or irregular bleeding when periods have become scanty.

## THE UTERUS

The menstrual cycle is often a good guide to a woman's well-being. Periods may be irregular during adolescence but usually settle into some sort of rhythm in the late teens. The sensitivity of the hypothalamus – and thus the pituitary – to mental state is shown by the fact that stress and depression can upset this cycle. A period can be brought on by a change in routine, such as a holiday, a house or job move or a wedding! Irregular bleeding can also result from illness, a gain or loss of weight or from excessive, strenuous exercise.

It may be difficult for you to assess whether your periods are 'normal', since our perception of our menstrual cycle is often affected by our expectations. Studies that have measured the amount of flow from women and then asked them for their own judgement have found that the same loss will be seen as excessive, average or light by different women. Similarly, while a regular but 'too frequent' flow may be normal for one woman, in another it could be a symptom of continuing stress or of inflammation.

Heavy bleeding can also be the result of stress and many adolescents find their periods are uncomfortably profuse until a rhythm has been established. It may, however, be a symptom of prolapse or fibroids, both conditions tending to appear in adult and older women. Prolapse is when the muscles and ligaments holding the uterus in place are weakened. The uterus and cervix may then slump downwards into the vagina. If the muscles of the vaginal wall are also affected, the organs can collapse down so far that part or all of the cervix protrudes out of the vagina. This is called procidentia. As well

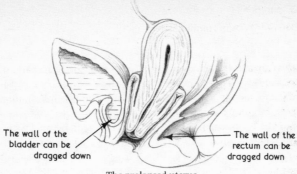

The wall of the
bladder can be
dragged down

The wall of the
rectum can be
dragged down

The prolapsed uterus

as heavy blood loss, symptoms of a prolapse include a dragging, full feeling, low backache and a difficulty in holding your water – incontinence. When you do pass water, you may find you have to return to the lavatory several times, to squeeze out a final few drops that will not come out immediately. Early signs can be a lump in the side of your vagina which disappears when you are lying down and gets bigger as your bladder fills.

Fibroids are bundles of fibrous tissue that can grow within the muscle of your uterus. They are not cancerous and so are not dangerous in themselves. As many as one in four women is likely to have fibroids, and they may grow without causing much trouble. They usually grow inside the wall of the uterus, when they are called intramural fibroids. Those growing on the outside of the womb are subserous fibroids and those in the lining of the womb are submucous fibroids. Submucous fibroids are the ones most likely to cause pain and heavy bleeding. They push out into the uterine cavity and expand the area of the lining of the womb, giving a greater surface to shed. Submucous fibroids can also extend on long stalks and when this happens, the uterus reacts as if it had a foreign body inside that needed to be expelled. The uterus will flex and contract, making periods longer, heavier and more painful. If the fibroid on its stalk is partly pushed out, it may jam the os and lead to constant pain and bleeding.

Subserous fibroids are often pain-free, but can grow large enough to press against the bowel or bladder, leading to difficulty in passing water or a movement. They may also grow out on stalks and sometimes the fibroid wraps around itself, cutting off blood supply. You

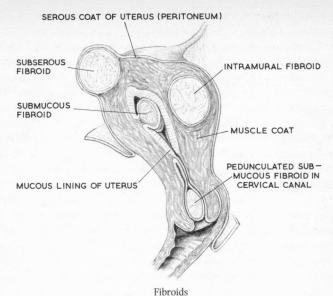

SEROUS COAT OF UTERUS (PERITONEUM)

SUBSEROUS
FIBROID

INTRAMURAL FIBROID

SUBMUCOUS
FIBROID

MUSCLE COAT

PEDUNCULATED SUB—
MUCOUS FIBROID IN
CERVICAL CANAL

MUCOUS LINING OF UTERUS

Fibroids

might then experience a sharp pain which recedes as the fibroid dies and hardens into what used to be called a 'womb stone'. Intramural fibroids are silent, unless they grow large enough to be noticeable, pushing on organs or giving you a pregnant or pot-belly appearance.

Unexpected bleeding can be a symptom of cancer, not only of the vagina or cervix but of the uterus. The most common cancer affecting the womb is cancer of the endometrium. This is more likely to occur in older women – the peak incidence is in the sixties – and is the reason why bleeding after the menopause should always, urgently, lead to a visit to a doctor. However, one in three cases do occur in women before menopause and women who are overweight or diabetic are particularly at risk. A quarter of women suffering from cancer of the uterus are pre-menopausal. Symptoms may include a brown, watery discharge and irregular bleeding. There may also be pain in the lower abdomen or belly, which is not severe but lasts for around one to two hours and tends to come at the same time each day.

The uterus may not always be the source of blood in a vaginal flow. As well as bleeding from an infected and inflamed cervix, you could experience some loss from a traumatized polyp. A polyp is a benign or non-cancerous growth of cells that is attached to the mucous membrane of the cervix. It can cause a watery discharge that may be bloodstained, and if it grows to some length may be dislodged or damaged by a tampon, finger or penis, and bleed.

Some blood that we may think has come from the vagina may actually be issuing from another source. It can be easy to see blood on our pants or on loo paper and make the obvious connection when, in fact, it is coming from the anus or rectum. Fissures – tiny splits in the skin around the anus – or haemorrhoids (piles) can both be the result of difficulty in passing solid waste. Piles are swollen veins that stick out as bumps or nodules around the anus or in the rectum, and can itch maddeningly and be scratched, or burst, until they bleed.

At times, the noticeable abnormality about periods is that they might be absent. The first, most obvious and most prevalent cause for periods not arriving is pregnancy! However unlikely and however unpleasant the consequences, if you are late, *always* suspect this first. If periods have never started by the age of eighteen, this is a cause for concern. It may be because of an imperforate hymen, when the maidenhead completely obstructs the vaginal opening and blood is flowing from the uterus but is unable to exit from the body. Disorders of the endocrine or hormone system which prevent maturity can be to blame, as can some specific diseases. Periods that have been established can be halted by drastic weight-change – gain or loss – by any stress that affects the hormone-releasing glands, or by disease or damage in them.

Abnormal bleeding may often be accompanied by pain in the back or lower belly. Most women do experience pain, either gripping and sudden or dull and prolonged, during their periods. This is caused by the uterus flexing and contracting in movements exactly like those that happen during childbirth. Instead of expelling a baby, the uterus acts to expel the lining of the womb. Some women also have pains low on one side of the belly some fourteen days before their next period. This is called Mittelschmerz or middle-pain, and is caused by the bursting of the follicle that expels a mature egg at ovulation. Some women also have a very slight amount of vaginal bleeding or 'spotting' at this time.

## THE PELVIC CAVITY

Vague abdominal pain could be a symptom of an ovarian cyst, or ovarian cancer. Ovarian cysts frequently cause very little trouble until they grow to a size where they press on other organs or cause discomfort during love-making. They can be painful, however, and they can burst, leaking into the pelvic cavity and causing serious infection. Ovarian cancer is most common in women in their sixties, but a sensible doctor will usually want to eliminate this when a middle-aged woman complains of discomfort in the abdomen and grumbling indigestion.

Prolapse can give rise to low backache, and acute or chronic cervicitis – infection of the cervix – can also lead to backache or pain in the lower belly. In cervicitis, examination or any movement of the cervix will hurt. Infections in the vagina, the cervix or the uterus can all lead to pain. Because the reproductive and waste-elimination organs in the pelvis lie so closely together, infection in one can spread to another. An infection can also lead to adhesions – scar tissue that accumulates around the site of an infection and can painfully immobilize an organ that should move freely, or stick it to another adjacent organ. Long-standing infections of the pelvic organs are known as PID – Pelvic Inflammatory Disease. PID can develop if sexually transmitted diseases (STDs) have been able to flourish without being detected or treated – chlamydia, which frequently is not diagnosed, or gonorrhoea which often shows no symptoms.

PID arises most in women with a history of having several sexual partners, since this places them at greater risk of contracting an STD, and in women who use the IUCD or coil for birth-control. This device can encourage infection, especially in women with multiple partners. If the fallopian tubes become infected, they may be blocked by scar tissue, making pregnancy difficult or impossible. The initial infection in PID, and PID in its early stages, may or may not be accompanied by the more obvious symptoms of a discharge, fever or pain. Chronic PID is more likely to show itself by a vague ill health and a pain which comes and goes. Often internal scar tissue is not obvious, even to an internal examination by a doctor. Symptoms may be dismissed by the sufferer or her medical advisers as 'just normal female pain and discomfort'. PID may only become apparent under a surgical examination, when the pelvis is opened and the adhesions can be seen.

Another illness that may be ignored or overlooked is endometriosis. In this, endometrial tissue – the cells that make up the lining of the womb – start growing outside the womb, usually on the surface of, or, less frequently, in the tissues of the pelvic organs such as the uterus, the ovaries, the bladder, the bowel and on the walls of the pelvic cavity. Endometrial tissue can also crop up in the vagina and in the navel, and it has a particular affinity for scar tissue. Just as in the womb, these cells build up and shed during the menstrual cycle, but since the resultant flow cannot find a convenient exit from the body, it forms cysts. These are called 'chocolate cysts' because of their dark appearance and syrupy interior. As well as pain, especially during menstruation and during intercourse, endometriosis often leads to tiredness and depression. It also produces an interesting 'catch-22' situation. A pregnancy can clear up the disease because the nine-month suspension of a normal menstrual cycle allows the rogue patches of endometrial tissue to decay and disappear. However, endometriosis can also affect your fertility, making it difficult to become pregnant in the first place.

Pain from problems in the pelvis may not seem to be located in the pelvis itself. As already mentioned, inflammation and infection can lead to low backache rather than a pain obviously coming from the cervix or uterus. Ectopic pregnancy (when a fertilized egg stops in the fallopian tube and starts developing into an embryo) will cause acute pain as it stretches and possibly bursts the tube, but not always in the abdomen. You may feel an ache just below the collar bone, instead of or as well as lower abdominal pain.

Alternatively, a pain that appears to come from the pelvis may actually be sited elsewhere. Irritable bowel syndrome can sometimes masquerade as painful periods or even endometriosis. In this condition, also sometimes known as spastic colon, the muscles in the intestine go into uncomfortable cramping spasms. You may experience swelling and a feeling of fullness as well as pain and have intermittent constipation and diarrhoea.

## BREASTS

Lumps in the breast probably cause far more alarm and distress than any other single symptom a woman might detect in her body. The immediate and obvious fear of any woman who finds a lump is that she has cancer. Breast cancer accounts for 20 per cent of all cancer deaths and is the leading cause of death in women aged forty to forty-five. It is, however, most likely to be found in women in their early sixties. One in seventeen women in the UK will be diagnosed as having breast cancer and of these one in three will die within two years. Most of these deaths are avoidable, as will be discussed in a later chapter. But any lump you discover is far *more* likely to be of a benign or innocent type. 50 per cent of women have these at some time or other.

Most women find their breasts become tender and swollen in the week before a period. Intermittent pain is far from uncommon, especially in teenagers, and is usually nothing to worry about. Furthermore, it is usual for breast tissue to become rubbery and lumpy under the surface before menstruation. Just as the uterus prepares for a pregnancy by building up a lining, so the breast adjusts to hormonal stimulus and makes itself ready to manufacture milk. Each month, if a pregnancy is not established, the tissue and fluid involved drain away, but the system is not as efficient as in the uterus. Tissue gradually builds up, and in women who delay or do not have a pregnancy, minor but uncomfortable problems can evolve. Lumpy breasts are also often found in women on the Pill.

Lumps under the surface can be a normal response to these monthly changes and if so are likely to build up and become most noticeable and tender in the second half of the menstrual cycle. This condition is called fibroadenosis or chronic cystic mastitis. Small cysts form in the breast tissue, which is itself fibrous, and these fill with fluid. Small cysts can cluster together forming a large lump, and individual cysts can grow quite large. These cysts, although sometimes painful, are benign and non-cancerous. Lumpiness from Pill-use or fibroadenosis is generally found in both breasts.

Cysts do not have to be associated with fibroadenosis, however, but can occur singly and in one breast when a duct becomes blocked for other reasons, and so can occur in women who have had early or several pregnancies. Single cysts may be less obviously painful than the multiplicity of nodules possible in fibroadenosis, but a large, painless lump could also suggest a benign tumour or fibroadenoma. This is a thickening and hardening of tissue, like a uterine fibroid, which can be a few inches in diameter. Not only are they painless, they are firm, regular and hard and appear to move freely under the skin when examined by hand. A single lump, of course, may indeed indicate a malignant tumour or cancer, and these can masquerade as fibroadenomas or hide behind them. Generally, malignant lumps are irregular in outline and tethered in place. This is why a breast lump, however seemingly innocent, should always be reported and watched. Cancerous lumps are rarely painful, so it is indeed possible to have fire without smoke.

There is no truth to the myth that a knock or other injury can cause cancer. Often, what does occur is that such an event can draw your attention to a previously unnoticed growth. However, there is some evidence to suggest that repeated trauma to a particular site might trigger delicate tissue to become cancerous. Most cancer of the breast occurs in the left side, and it has even been suggested by medical experts that the fact that most men are right-handed is not unrelated.

## NIPPLES

Breast problems can also show themselves by affecting the nipples. It is perfectly normal for nipples to lie flat and relaxed except when stimulated, and it is not uncommon for women to have inverted nipples – nipples which vanish into a dimple instead of coming erect. If this occurs at puberty, it is not a symptom of any underlying disease. It can, however, be annoying to a young woman who then feels she seems less attractive and sexually responsive than the norm, and it can make later breastfeeding difficult. However, if a previously 'upfront' nipple suddenly draws inwards, especially if you are nearing menopause or beyond, it might well suggest the presence of a tumour or other underlying condition.

Apart from breast lumps, the most important symptom to watch for in your breasts is a discharge from the nipple. It is not uncommon for women to be able to express a white, milky discharge, even when they are not pregnant or breastfeeding. Sometimes, but rarely, this can be an indication of a tumour or of disease in a hormone-producing

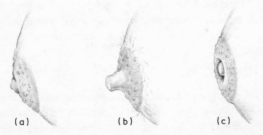

(a)      (b)      (c)

The nipple in *a* resting, *b* stimulated and *c* indrawn states gland. More often, it is a reaction to some common drugs such as those given for depression and high blood-pressure or, more frequently, the Combined oral contraceptive pill. Frequent manipulation of the breasts in love-play can also stimulate milk production. Breast milk can be produced for years after childbirth, as long as stimulation continues, which is why women could – and in parts of the world still do – earn their living as 'wet nurses'. However, if a discharge is bloody, straw-coloured or clear or pus-streaked, then it certainly needs medical investigation.

During puberty, girls might find their breasts exude a clear liquid, as well as being red and tender, and at this time such a discharge is normal. After puberty, it could suggest a cyst. Benign lesions can also lead to a bloody flow, ranging from pink to red or brown/black. A bloody discharge might be a symptom of a malignant tumour, however. Tumours, both benign and malignant, can also set off a foul-looking greenish, blackish discharge – though this is far more likely to be a symptom of fibroadenosis. A pus-stained discharge can be the result of mastitis – an infection that normally occurs during breastfeeding as the result of a milk duct becoming blocked. An abcess can develop, causing pain and a general feeling of ill health.

Occasionally, the sebaceous or oil-producing glands surrounding the nipples become infected. This is particularly likely to happen during breastfeeding, when they are large and prominent. A pus-stained discharge from this source may be mistaken for one coming from the nipple. A form of cancer, called Paget's disease, can also set off soreness and itching in the nipples and lead them to crack and weep.

Breast cancer causes more deaths and mutilating operations in women than other forms of reproductive cancer because, frequently, a malignant tumour is small, painless and far enough below the surface of the breast not to be felt by a hand examination. It may be found in other ways, however, and these will be discussed in later chapters.

## GENERAL SYMPTOMS

There is a sexually transmitted disease that makes itself felt through several symptoms rather than attacking the sexual organs themselves. This is AIDS – acquired immune deficiency syndrome. The syndrome is not in itself a disease. What happens is that a virus, known as HIV or HTLV 3, can be passed from an infected person to a contact, via blood or body fluids. So far, most people found to have the virus in the Western world have belonged to a limited number of groups. These are male homosexuals, intravenous drug abusers who have shared needles, haemophiliacs in receipt of infected transfusions, the sexual contacts of any of these and babies born to infected mothers. However, it is more useful to think in terms of high-risk behaviour than high-risk populations. Non-sexual contact and some intimate behaviour with an infected person is safe, and not everyone belonging to these groups either has the virus or is at risk of catching it. But since you cannot tell by looking at them or even knowing them that a partner is one of these or uninfected, the best option is to avoid certain practices rather than try to avoid certain groups of people!

The virus works by damaging the body's own immune system. Not everyone who is infected by the virus goes on to develop the syndrome. A person who does so may find themselves suffering from one or a number of 'opportunistic' infections. These take the leeway granted by the lapse in efficiency of the body's defence against disease to strike and are likely to be one of a few, quite rare conditions. The symptoms that might suggest you had AIDS would be:

- a feeling of constant tiredness that has gone on for some weeks with no apparent cause;
- a sudden weight-loss of more than ten pounds over a couple of months, with no dieting;
- a fever, and sweating at night;
- breathlessness and a hoarse, dry cough lasting for several weeks;
- swollen glands in the neck or armpits;
- patches of bruised-looking skin, pink or purple, that persist and get larger instead of fading.

There are other conditions related to the reproductive system that are felt throughout your body, rather than focusing on one area. A disorder in any of the hormone-producing glands may make you feel tired, depressed and unwell. However, most women react at some time in their lives to the ebb and flow of hormones that both trigger and respond to the menstrual cycle. A range of symptoms of varying intensity and discomfort can surround menstruation. In the week before bleeding, you may experience tiredness, tension, depression and irritability. You may find it difficult to concentrate and become forgetful, you may find it difficult to sleep, feel sick, dizzy, suffer aches and pains, headaches and cold sweats. You may also find your stomach bloats, your fingers and ankles swell and your breasts feel sore and tender. This collection of problems is called pre-menstrual syndrome (PMS) or pre-menstrual tension (PMT). Whether you classify PMS as a disorder, or see it as something that is part of being a woman, might depend on many factors. These will be discussed in the next chapter.

## CONDITIONS THAT MAY AFFECT THE GENITALS —— AND REPRODUCTIVE ORGANS ——

### Amenorrhoea

What is it?    Absence of periods.

Symptom:    No periods.

Causes:    Adolescence. It is quite normal for periods to be irregular in the first two years of menstruation.
Pregnancy.
Drastic weight-change – loss or gain.
Breastfeeding.
Childbirth.
Coming off the Combined contraceptive pill.
Stress.
Illness.
Certain medicines.
Diabetes or a thyroid disorder.
Menopause.

Action:    See your doctor, who may offer treatment, recommend that you wait and see or take some action yourself.

### Cancer of the genital tract, cervix or vagina

What is it?    Malignant tumour in the vagina or the neck of the uterus.

Symptoms:    No obvious symptoms in the early stages, although this condition can be picked up by a simple test – the Pap or Smear test – that spots the changes that come *before* cancer develops.

Offensive discharge – bloodstained or watery.
Irregular bleeding – especially after menopause.

Causes:       Although not *causes*, certain factors are associated with this disease, such as smoking, early unprotected intercourse, early motherhood, a history of STDs and a sexual relationship with a partner with a history of STDs.

Women whose mothers were given diethylstilbestrol (DES) during pregnancy to treat threatened miscarriage are particularly prone to vaginal cancer.

Action:       See your doctor immediately.

### Cancer of the endometrium

What is it?       Malignant tumour in the lining of the womb.

Symptoms:       Often asymptomatic, especially in early stages. Irregular bleeding, especially after menopause. Offensive, bloodstained watery discharge.

Causes:       After menopause, the use of artificial oestrogen without the addition of progestogen can increase risks.

Action:       See your doctor immediately.

### Cancer of the ovary

What is it?       Malignant tumour on one of the egg-cases.

Symptoms:       Often asymptomatic in early stages. Pain or discomfort and 'indigestion'.

Action:       See your doctor immediately.

### Cancer of the breast

What is it?       Malignant tumour in the breast.

Symptoms:       Hard lump or area of dimpled skin. Itching round nipple.

Discharge from nipple – bloodstained, green or blackish.

Inward drawing of nipple.

Action:       See your doctor immediately.

## Chlamydia

| | |
|---|---|
| What is it? | STD that affects the vagina and cervix. |
| Symptoms: | Offensive greyish-white discharge. |
| | Pus-stained mucus in cervical os. |
| | Pain. |
| | Cervix inflamed and liable to bleed. |
| Causes: | A difficult-to-trace, sexually transmitted organism. |
| Action: | See your doctor as soon as possible. |

**Crabs** See **Pubic lice.**

## Cystitis

| | |
|---|---|
| What is it? | An inflammatory infection of the bladder. |
| Symptoms: | Pain or burning sensation on passing water. Cloudy, dark or bloodstained urine. |
| | Urge to pass water even when bladder is empty. |
| | Fever. |
| | Pain. |
| Causes: | Infection by bacteria of the urethra climbing into the bladder. Can also happen from obstruction or deformity in the bladder. |
| Action: | Take self-help measures outlined in Chapter 4. If it persists, see your doctor. |

## Cysts (breasts)

| | |
|---|---|
| What is it? | A fluid-filled sac in the breast tissue. |
| Symptoms: | One or several hard round lumps in one or both breasts. |
| | Pain. |
| | Clear discharge from nipple. |
| Cause: | Duct becomes blocked and resultant sac fills with fluid and presses against surrounding tissue. |
| Action: | See your doctor, in case the lump is actually a tumour. Doctor may then advise you to let it resolve. |

## Dysmenorrhoea

| | |
|---|---|
| What is it? | Period pain. There are two types – primary and secondary. |

*Primary*

| | |
|---|---|
| Symptoms: | Present from menarche or early in adolescence. Tiredness, tension, headaches and nausea. |
| | Gripping pain on day before period starts – usually relieved by flow and often disappears with maturity, after pregnancy or if sufferer takes the oral contraceptive pill. |
| Causes: | Emotional or hormonal imbalance. |

*Secondary*

| | |
|---|---|
| Symptoms: | Develops after a history of normal periods. Pain, headaches, nausea, tension and tiredness. |
| Causes: | Emotional; or fibroids, endometriosis, polyps, inflammation in the womb, tumours. |
| Action: | See your doctor who may offer treatment or suggest that you self-treat, as explained in Chapter 4. |

### Ectopic pregnancy

| | |
|---|---|
| What is it? | A pregnancy that occurs outside the womb, usually in a fallopian tube. |
| Symptoms: | Pain in lower abdomen and/or below collarbone. Amenorrhoea, but not always. |
| | Collapse due to rupturing of tube. |
| Causes: | Scar tissue or blockage in a tube due to infection, or lack of movement in cilia lining tube. |
| | A history of PID or the use of an IUCD increases risk. |
| Action: | See your doctor – urgently. |

### Endometriosis

| | |
|---|---|
| What is it? | Tissue that normally lines the womb grows elsewhere in the pelvic cavity, especially on scar tissue. |
| Symptoms: | Pain and tenderness, especially around menstruation or during intercourse. |
| | Depression. |
| | Tiredness. |
| Action: | See your doctor. |

### Erosions

| | |
|---|---|
| What is it? | Red and roughened areas of surface of cervix. |

Symptoms:     Often asymptomatic.
Increase in vaginal lubrication.
If inflamed, an offensive and bloodstained discharge.

Causes:     Cells lining cervical os extend on to surface of the cervix during puberty, after pregnancy, during Pill use or as woman matures.

Action:     See your doctor who may offer treatment or advise you to let it resolve.

### Fibroadenoma

What is it?     Benign tumour in breast, composed of hard fibrous tissue.

Symptom:     Single hard lump in one breast. Painless and often only discovered by accident or by examination. Lump is often round and appears to move freely under the skin.

Action:     See your doctor.

### Fibroadenosis (also called chronic cystis mastitis)

What is it?     Condition which occurs in many women, especially those who do not have or delay pregnancy, or older women.

Symptoms:     Lumpy or rubbery masses or a single lump in one or both breasts.
Pain, tenderness and swelling, especially in the second half of the menstrual cycle.

Cause:     Reaction to hormones.

Action:     See your doctor and then, on advice, leave to resolve or self-treat.

### Fibroids

What is it?     Growth of fibrous tissue in the walls of the uterus.

Symptoms:     May be asymptomatic.
Heavy, irregular and painful bleeding.
Dragging, 'bearing down' sensation.
Infertility.

Interference with urination and bowel movements if mass presses down on bladder or bowel.

Cause:    Probably hormonal.

Action:    See your doctor.

## Galactorrhoea

What is it?    Milk produced by the breasts outside the normal range of pregnancy and breastfeeding.

Symptoms:    A milky discharge from the breasts.

Causes:    Persistent stimulation of the breasts, Combined Pill use or a disorder of the hormone-producing glands.

Action:    See your doctor and, after advice, leave to resolve.

## Genital warts

What is it?    Growths on the genitals. They can be small and smooth or large and fleshy.

Symptoms:    If internal, there may be no sign. Can bleed if torn by intercourse, examination or tampon use.

Cause:    Virus, usually passed on by sexual contact.

Action:    See a doctor.

## Gonorrhoea

What is it?    Sexually transmitted disease.

Symptoms:    Can be asymptomatic until the development of PID (see further).
Burning sensation on passing water.
Vaginal discharge.
Pain in lower abdomen.
Occasionally discharge and itching in anus.

Causes:    Bacteria passed, usually during sexual contact, but *might* survive for short time in warm, moist conditions – on shared wash flannel.

Action:    See a doctor.

**Haemorrhoids** (piles)

What is it?    Swollen veins in walls of the back passage or near the
                    entrance to the anus.

Symptoms:      Pain.
                    Bleeding.
                    Itching.

Causes:        Straining to pass a bowel motion. A bad diet with little
                    fibre. Lack of exercise, frequent use of laxatives and
                    pregnancy can also be contributing factors.

Action:        See your doctor and/or self-treat.

**Herpes**

What is it?    Painful cold sores on genitals.

Symptoms:      May be asymptomatic if sores are internal and
                    unseen.
                    Itching, tingling sensation followed by formation of
                    small blisters – singly or in groups.
                    Sometimes fever, swollen glands and flu-like symp-
                    toms.
                    Pain or burning on passing water.

Causes:        Virus transferred by intimate contact. After initial
                    attack, virus becomes dormant and either does not
                    reappear or causes symptoms again in response to
                    physical stimulation such as friction or heat, or emo-
                    tional stimulation such as stress, pre-menstruation
                    or if carrier is generally below par.

Action:        See your doctor. In the case of repeat attacks, you may
                    also have to self-treat.

**'Honeymoon' cystitis**

What is it?    Inflammation of the urethra or urethritis.

Symptoms:      Discomfort, pain or a burning sensation on passing
                    water.

Causes:        Friction from sexual intercourse or the introduction of
                    bacteria into the urethra.

Action:            Self-treat on first symptoms, as outlined in Chapter 4.
                   If it persists, see your doctor.

## Mastitis

What is it?        Infection in the breast that can lead to abscess.

Symptoms:          Tenderness in breast followed by a feeling of fullness
                   and hard swelling.

Causes:            Bacteria entering breast, usually through a crack in
                   the nipple during breastfeeding.

Action:            See your doctor.

## Mittelschmerz

What is it?        Pain midway between periods.

Symptoms:          Aching or sharp pain in lower abdomen.
                   Spots of blood from the vagina.

Causes:            Rupturing of follicle on ovary as egg is released.

Action:            See your doctor who may treat you or advise you to
                   let it resolve.

## Non-specific genital infections

What is it?        General catch-all title given to infections in the urethra
                   (urethritis) and the vagina (vaginitis) where the
                   specific organism causing the inflammation is diffi-
                   cult to trace.

Symptoms:          Pain and inflammation in the genital area.
                   Pain and burning on passing water.
                   Urge to pass water.
                   Discharge from the vagina.

Causes:            Various bacteria introduced by sexual contact or by
                   sufferer herself.

Action:            See a doctor.

## Ovarian cysts

What is it?        Fluid-filled or solid sac that forms on the ovary.

Symptoms:          Often asymptomatic.
                   Pain or tenderness in lower abdomen.
                   Pain during intercourse.

Causes:      Often a follicle which has not ruptured to release an egg. Can be a developmental fault.

Action:      See your doctor.

### Pelvic inflammatory disease (PID)

What is it?   Widespread and long-term infection in the reproductive and pelvic organs.

Symptoms:    Often asymptomatic.
             In acute cases, high fever and severe pain.
             In chronic cases, grumbling pain and ill health.
             Infertility.

Causes:      Infection in the uterus, fallopian tubes and other organs in the pelvic cavity, e.g. the appendix.
             Infection from untreated STD. The condition is more likely in women with multiple sexual partners or who use an IUCD.
             Botched abortion – i.e. illegal or 'backstreet' abortion.

Action:      See a doctor.

### Polyps

What is it?   Benign tumour or growth found on the cervix or in the vagina.

Symptoms:    Watery discharge.
             Blood in discharge, especially after intercourse.

Causes:      Unknown.

Action:      See your doctor who may treat you or advise you to let it resolve.

### Pre-menstrual syndrome (PMS or PMT)

What is it?   Collection of uncomfortable changes that many women experience in the week or so before menstruation.

Symptoms:    Depression, irritation, tiredness.
             Insomnia, headaches, aches and pains.
             Tender and swollen breasts, bloated stomach.
             Nausea, inability to concentrate, clumsiness.

| Causes: | Hormonal fluctuations. |
| Action: | See your doctor and/or self-treat as outlined in Chapter 4. |

### Prolapse

| What is it? | Collapse of the uterus and cervix downwards into the vagina. |
| Symptoms: | Urge to pass water frequently and difficulty in holding back. |
| | Uncomfortable feeling of 'bearing down' and heaviness. |
| | Lump in vagina which goes away when lying down. |
| | Backache. |
| Causes: | Weakness in pelvic ligaments and/or vaginal muscles. |
| Action: | See your doctor. |

### Pubic lice (crabs)

| What is it? | Infestation by small insects. |
| Symptoms: | Itching and rash in pubic area. |
| | Small objects stuck on to pubic hair. These are the nits or egg cases. |
| Causes: | Passed by intimate contact with infected person. |
| Action: | See a doctor or self-treat as outlined in Chapter 4. |

### Syphilis

| What is it? | Sexually transmitted disease that can be fatal if left untreated. |
| Symptoms: | Stage 1: Painful sore in genital area. |
| | Stage 2: Fever, headache, sore throat, and rash appearing anywhere on body. |
| | Stage 3: Severe, permanent damage to heart, brain and other vital organs. |
| Cause: | Organism passed by sexual contact with infected person. |
| Action: | See a doctor. |

### Thrush

| What is it? | Yeast infection affecting vagina or vulva. |

Symptoms:    Itching and possibly pain and swelling in vulva.
             Thick, white, yeasty-smelling vaginal discharge.
             Discomfort on passing water.

Causes:      Can be passed by intimate contact, or on towels or
             flannels, but most frequently arises spontaneously.
             The thrush organism usually lives harmlessly inside
             us and only becomes troublesome if it multiplies.
             This happens if the moisture in the vagina becomes
             too alkaline, through pregnancy, illness, bad diet or
             through being interfered with.

Action:      See a doctor and/or self-treat as outlined in Chapter 4.

**Toxic shock syndrome** (TSS)

What is it?   Unusual infection related to tampon-use.

Symptoms:    Sore throat and high fever.
             Rash on skin.
             Muscle pains and diarrhoea.

Causes:      Infection by bacteria through damage to vaginal walls
             or by contaminated tampons. Found when super-
             absorbent tampons (now withdrawn) used or if
             tampon left inside too long (tampons should be chan-
             ged at least three times a day).
             Damage to vagina by fingernail, tampon inserter tube
             or dirtied tampon.

Action:      See your doctor.

**Trichomoniasis** (trich or TV)

What is it?   Infection of vagina and urethra.

Symptoms:    Foul, itchy or sore yellow or white vaginal discharge.

Cause:       Parasite usually passed by sexual contact.

Action:      See a doctor.

# CHAPTER 3

# Examination Techniques

W*hy* should you regularly examine your breasts or genitals or ask a professional to do so? Surely the procedure is uncomfortable, messy and embarrassing? Surely you would rather not know whether anything was amiss, since little can be done anyway, especially if the disorder is something such as cancer?

These are the beliefs behind many women's reluctance to have regular internal and breast examinations or to screen their own bodies. None are – or need to be – true.

For a start, much of our discomfort and embarrassment is caused by misinformation and a lack of real knowledge about these parts of our bodies. If our bodies were genuinely familiar to us – a lifelong friend rather than a stranger – we could feel comfortable and appreciative rather than critical and uneasy at their shapes, textures and odours. If we had more confidence about ourselves, we would probably find intimate examinations, by a doctor or by ourselves, less distasteful and intimidating. Far from being a waste of time, early diagnosis of any unusual condition could be a life saver.

There are many problems, both minor and major, that can be detected by you or by a professional and be easily dealt with before they take a serious hold. Some of these, if ignored, can cause you major damage and discomfort. Many cancers CAN BE CURED – but they *must* be caught at an early stage for this to be possible. At present, one in three women diagnosed as having breast cancer dies within two years. But this is because breast cancer is almost invariably only found in its advanced stages. It has been estimated that screening could reduce deaths from breast cancer by 40 per cent. A Swedish study has shown that regular breast X-rays reduced deaths from this disease by a third in a group of over-fifty year olds.

Some conditions can only be found by a doctor using sophisticated equipment or tests. But most of the conditions we have mentioned are far from 'silent'. They make themselves known in subtle ways as they slowly become worse. A woman who is aware of how her body feels, looks and smells in a healthy state, will notice early signs, and be able to take steps to return to health herself, or ask for advice and help. 90 per cent of women who are found to have *advanced* cancer of the cervix have never had a smear test.

## THE MEDICAL EXAMINATION

The internal and breast examination can be alarming and confusing if you have no idea what it is that the doctor is looking for or trying to do. The equipment necessary to get the best results can also be intimidating, if you have no idea of its function.

Many women are embarrassed even at the thought of an intimate examination, let alone the reality. Doctors are used to women apologizing – for the appearance, smell or general condition of their genitals. We are often brought up to consider 'down there' not only to be a taboo area, but one that is unsavoury or unhygienic. There is no need to apologize. Vulvas come in all shapes and sizes, and each is beautiful in its own way. The moisture and wrinkles in your genital area all have a function and are meant to be there, so you have nothing of which to be ashamed. Washing too vigorously soon before an intimate examination and douching the morning before can, in fact, be a positive hindrance to a health check. If you have a troublesome discharge, washing will remove vital evidence. If you are worried about the amount and texture of your vaginal lubrication or the moistness on your labia, washing it off beforehand can hardly help the doctor make a decision as to whether it is normal or the symptom of a problem. The odour of a discharge is often a vital part of diagnosis. Thrush, for instance, has a distinct yeasty smell, while a fishy odour could suggest an infection from the organism Gardnerella vaginalis. The colour is also important as a guide to diagnosis.

Unless your specific query or worry is about your periods, it is usually unwise to have an internal examination and smear test during menstruation or within three days of your period finishing. This is *not* because the flow is in any way unpleasant or dangerous, or would upset or disgust the doctor. It is because the flow may hide or mask other symptoms that should be followed up, or confuse any interpretation of the test.

Before you go in for your examination, check with the doctor or another member of staff whether you will need to give a urine sample. A full bladder during the examination would be acutely uncomfortable for you and get in the way of any investigation the doctor is trying to make! Empty yourself, but do so into the container they will give you, if this is required.

A screening examination can be done by a doctor or a nurse. In some health centres or surgeries the tests may be shared between both. For convenience, I shall refer to the examining professional throughout the next section as 'the doctor'.

## WEIGHT AND BLOOD-PRESSURE

Before asking you to strip off, most doctors will take two measurements – your weight and your blood pressure. Both are important as indicators of present and future health. Having your weight within a specific range for your age, height and build is nothing to do with vanity. Small and slim is not necessarily beautiful and there is also nothing necessarily unattractive in the more Rubenesque body. You have every right to object to a society that insists on women being skinny clothes-horses. You should, however, be aware that being either over- or underweight can be a threat to your well-being. Being underweight can throw the body's hormonal system into disarray. As the body's essential stores of fat melt away, periods become irregular or even cease, resistance to disease may be impaired and the digestive system could be damaged. If you carry excess weight, the main effect is that your heart and circulatory system will come under strain. The heart has to pump harder to push your blood around your body, and in doing so will become weakened. Your arteries are likely to thicken, increasing your risk of thrombosis or blood clots. Extra weight can also add to the wear and tear on joints and increases the risks of your developing osteoarthritis. Obesity is linked with a higher risk of diabetes – and both with a higher instance of endometrial cancer. If you are overweight, the chances are that you are not enjoying a healthy lifestyle with a good diet and regular exercise, both of which are essential for the maintenance of good health.

Having checked your weight, the doctor will want to find out how hard your heart is working. He does so by taking your blood-pressure. Blood-pressure is measured with a sphygmomanometer: this consists of an inflatable cuff attached to a measuring device – either an electronic scale or a mercury column like a thermometer. The cuff is

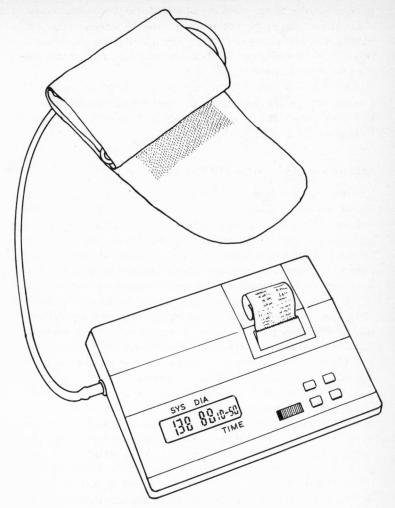

Digital sphygmomanometer

wrapped around an arm and inflated. The doctor listens for the point at which your circulation is stopped and the sound of the blood pumping ceases. The pressure it takes to do this is thus equal to the pressure your heart is exerting to pump blood out. This is called the systolic pressure. The cuff is then deflated and the doctor listens for

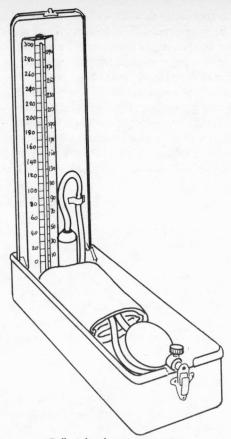

Bulb-style sphygmomanometer

the sound of blood returning. When this is heard, it is recorded on the measuring device – this is the diastolic pressure.

In overweight or stressed people, or those with clogged arteries, the pump obviously has to work particularly strongly to push the blood-supply around the system. If you are trying to water the garden, think of how much you have to increase the amount coming from the tap if someone stands on the hosepipe. This shows in the readings. Blood-pressure is expressed by writing systolic over diastolic. Most adults would have a systolic pressure of around 100 to 140, and a diastolic of between 60 and 90. 120/70 is a fairly average figure, therefore, for a reasonably fit adult woman, although a young, slim woman may be 90/60 and still be healthy. Blood pressure rises as you grow older and you might expect an increase of around 5 points in 10 years as you begin ageing. Roughly speaking, your systolic pressure is equivalent to your age plus 100.

Blood-pressure is the measure of the force it takes to push your blood around your body. This is distinct from your pulse, which is the measure of frequency or how often the heart beats in a minute. Our average woman, with a blood-pressure of 120/70 may, for instance, also have a pulse of 80 beats a minute. If she was very fit, it may be as low as 70 or even 65, without changing her blood-pressure.

## THE 'INTERNAL'

These tests completed, you would be asked to remove clothing covering your bottom half and to lie down on a couch. In some cases, this may have 'stirrups'. These are two devices on either side of the couch, over which you drape your legs at the calf or knee. The doctor can then stand or sit at the end of the couch, in between your spread legs, with a good, unobstructed view of your vulva.

Most doctors now realize that couches with stirrups make women feel extraordinarily exposed and vulnerable. You are not exactly tied down, but it certainly feels less easy to extricate yourself from the stirrups than just to close your knees together while lying on an ordinary couch. However much you may want to be co-operative and allow the doctor to look at you, it does make you feel better if you can have the *control* to stop the examination when you want. Having a finger on a panic button often ensures that you never use it, but not having access to one certainly makes you feel like panicking. So if your doctor uses a couch with stirrups and you find this unpleasant, say that you would rather not use them. Having lain down on the couch, you would be asked to bend your knees, lay your feet flat on the couch and allow your legs to relax and open.

The doctor will first look at your vulva. The aspects considered might be: is there any evidence of rash or irritation? Are the labia plump and a healthy pink and is the hair-growth thin and scanty or within a normal range? Are there any growths such as warts or polyps, or any sores?

Having looked at your external genitals, the doctor will probably move on to the internal. Nobody *enjoys* having an internal, but if you can lay aside your shyness and control your fears of being invaded, the experience is *not* painful. The muscles around the vagina are surprisingly powerful. They are supposedly under your conscious control, so that just as you can concentrate and clamp shut or release the muscles around the urethra to stop or start a flow of water, so you can clench or relax those around the vagina. However, if you feel nervous, you may well find it difficult to stay relaxed and you could find the muscles almost go into spasm. Although the flexible tube that is the vagina is well able to stretch, painlessly, to accommodate anything a doctor would need to introduce, having to contend against rigid muscles could make the experience uncomfortable or even painful for you.

The doctor will put on surgical gloves, which are disposable and plastic. This is *not* because you or any of your body fluids are unpleasant or dirty. Mostly it is to protect *you* from being contaminated by any germs on his or her hands. It is difficult to ensure that hands are completely sterile and free from harmful material in any ordinary doctor's surgery, but these gloves, carefully packed in airtight containers, can guarantee your safety. You need not fear catching anything from a previous patient, and if you do have an infection there is no chance of its being passed on.

The first action he or she is likely to take is gently to part the labia and look at the vaginal opening, to check whether there is any sign of a problematical discharge and that the area is a healthy colour. The doctor may then insert one finger inside, just to check that there are no obstructions, either through a degree of vaginismus or through your having forgotten to take out a tampon.

A speculum will then be inserted. This is an instrument made of plastic or metal. It is designed to gently hold apart the walls of the vagina, which are usually held collapsed shut and touching each other. The speculum is made up of two long, flat, scoop-shaped bowls, hinged at the end in a ring. It looks rather like a duck's bill. Kind and sensible professionals make sure it is warm before trying to insert it – especially if the device is metal and the day is cold! A dab of lubricating cream is often placed on the end to make insertion easier, unless a 'smear' test is going to be done. Cream would affect the result of this, so it is not used. With the bills held closed, the end of the speculum is inserted into the vagina and gently eased in until the hinged end comes up flat against the vulva. The hinge is then operated and the spoon ends move apart gently, pushing aside the vaginal walls. This

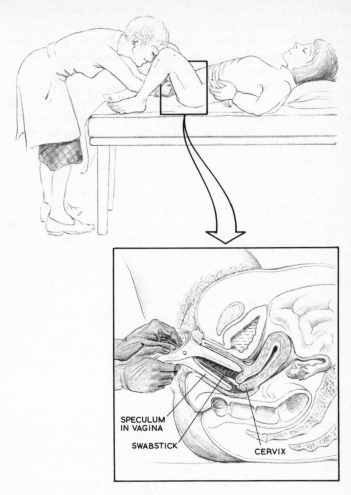

SPECULUM
IN VAGINA

SWABSTICK

CERVIX

Doctor taking a smear

brings the end of your vagina, the cervix and the length of the vagina
into clear view. Your cervix can then be examined for any signs of
abnormal discharge or for erosions. The colour of the cervix and
vagina can be checked, and any signs of infection, damage or growths
can be looked at.

## THE SMEAR TEST

A Pap (Papanicolaou or smear) test will then be taken, when a few cells are collected from the surface of the cervix. The name comes from Dr George Papanicolaou, the inventor of this test and thus the benefactor of womankind! Cells are collected by rubbing the shaped end of a wooden spatula across the cervix. This is not painful as the covering does not have to be scraped violently to make some cells come away. If you think of what happens when you wash yourself in a bath or shower with a cloth, you will remember that rolls of what might appear to be dirt come loose. These are in fact layers of dead skin, and since our bodies are in a constant state of renewing, it is very easy to gather up shed cells from any surface. These cells are smeared on to a glass slide and the result is doused in a liquid to 'fix' or preserve it. The slide is then sent away to a specialized laboratory, usually in a local hospital, for examination. The doctor may also use a pipette, or thin glass tube, or a cotton-tipped applicator to gather secretions from the top of the vagina or from the cervical canal.

The principle of smear tests is that cells have one appearance when healthy but change when they are inflamed, cancerous, or preparing to become cancerous. Long before an obvious tumour develops, these changes can be seen at cell level under a microscope and action can be taken. The laboratory examination can show whether the cells collected in your smear test or swab came from the cervix or have been shed from the vagina or endometrium.

The process by which cells change from healthy to cancerous is usually fairly slow. A smear test will alert your doctor to the fact that *something* is wrong, but this may not mean that the something is necessarily cancer or is going to become cancer. If your test comes back marked 'abnormal', there are several possibilities.

The abnormality noticed could be benign or innocent. It could have been an unsatisfactory smear. If there was too much blood or pus in the sample, it may have been difficult to see anything else. Too few cells could have been collected, or the 'fixing' process may have failed to preserve the cells. It could be that you have 'inflammatory changes'. These may indicate infection with wart or herpes virus, or infection by an organism such as trichomoniasis, candida, chlamydia or gonorrhoea.

Alternatively, the smear could show what are known as 'neoplastic abnormalities', which means an abnormal formation of new tissue.

The laboratory report may contain some terms to describe what is going on, while your doctor may use other words to say the same thing.

The smear might have found 'glandular tissue'. This would mean that cells from the uterus had been detected. This can happen if you had your smear done soon after your period, or can be caused by the action of a coil or IUCD, if you have one. The doctor would want to do a follow-up test to make sure that what it did *not* indicate was pre-cancerous or cancerous changes in the uterus.

The smear might show 'cervical intraepithelial neoplasia' (CIN) or abnormal growth in the covering of the cervix. There are three grades of CIN smears: CIN1, or very mild or mild dysplasia, also known as mild dyskaryosis; CIN2 or moderate dysplasia, also known as moderate dyskaryosis; CIN3, or severe dysplasia, also known as severe dyskaryosis. Finally, the smear might show malignant cells or invasive cancer.

It is not uncommon to have a CIN1 smear, and in most cases – about 60 per cent – the cells revert to normal on their own. For this reason, the discovery of a CIN1 smear is not in itself a cause for panic, and the usual response to it is to schedule another smear in three months, to see whether the dysplasia has progressed or retreated. If you see that a smear of yours has come back marked 'abnormal cells found', do *not* assume that you have cancer or anything necessarily to worry about. Equally, if the doctor treating you does not send you for immediate treatment, do not assume that they are being negligent.

Moderate or severe dysplasia will need further examination. If this is diagnosed in a smear of yours, you are likely to be sent for a colposcopy. A colposcope is a specialized instrument that enables a doctor to take a closer look at the surface of the cervix and vagina. They are available in some hospitals and clinics. The area to be examined is often painted with a dye and abnormal cells show up by not taking the stain. When identified, the worrying cells can be removed – either by cauterizing or burning them, freezing them away, or evaporating them with a laser. Cells can also be removed for further examination – a punch biopsy. If the doctor suspects that more than just surface cells are involved, a cone biopsy could be advised. In this, a cone-shaped area of surface and deeper tissue is taken to see if the cell changes have begun to work down.

Carcinoma is said to be present or *in situ* when there is a clump of abnormal cells which are malignant and capable of spreading or metastasizing. This is the first stage of cancer. The second stage is the micro-invasive, when cancer cells are beginning to break off and migrate to set up colonies elsewhere. The third stage is the invasive, when this process is well under way. A cone biopsy may be diagnostic – to find out what is happening – or may be the treatment itself, to remove all the affected cells. This is sufficient in CIN smears, and would be followed up by regular smears and possibly colposcopies to make sure the treatment has worked.

If you have not yet completed your family, it may be worthwhile discussing whether such treatment should be done by laser rather than conventional surgery. If the area of tissue to be excised is significant, surgery could leave you with an 'incompetent' cervix – one that would have difficulty in remaining closed during a pregnancy and which would thus put you at risk of having a miscarriage. Lasers are, unfortunately, expensive and your local hospital may not have one. Your doctor is able to refer you to any treatment centre in the UK, not just your local hospital, but waiting-lists for both colposcopes and lasers are often long. You may even feel it worth the money to go privately for such treatment. Micro-invasive cancer may also only need cone biopsy, but could lead to a hysterectomy or removal of the womb and surrounding tissue. Invasive cancer will probably lead to a mixture of surgery, radiotherapy and chemotherapy, depending on the age of the woman and the extent of the malignancy.

## THE BI-MANUAL

After taking a smear, the doctor will remove the speculum, holding it open so as not to pinch delicate tissue. A 'bi-manual' or two-handed examination will then be done. With one hand, he or she will first feel inside your vagina, to make sure there are no abnormal or unusual lumps or bumps. Vaginal tumours, for instance, may show as a painless lump in the side wall. He or she may feel for the Bartholin's Glands, which are two pea-shaped and -sized glands on either side of the entrance to your vagina that can usually be felt only if they are infected or have cysts. Finally, the tips of the fingers will feel for the cervix and stabilize it. The second hand will then be placed on your lower abdomen or belly. By pressing together, your pelvic organs can be felt between the two hands. If you can imagine feeling around inside a cloth bag while wearing gloves, and trying to identify your

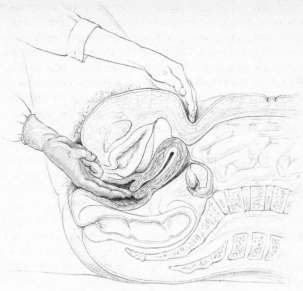

Doctor making a bi-manual examination

wallet, keys and make-up bag, you can understand what the doctor is trying to do. Through the walls of the vagina, your uterus and ovaries can be felt and moved. The doctor can tell whether there are any problems by feeling if the organs move as freely as they should, and by whether they feel their characteristic shapes, sizes and textures. The fallopian tubes are usually too slender and pliable to be felt easily, unless they are blocked by scar tissue or infection, in which case, they too will become palpable or capable of being felt. Any pain you feel during what should *not* be a painful experience will tell the doctor if there is anything amiss.

In some cases, the doctor may do a rectal examination – putting a finger into the rectum or waste passage. There can be two reasons for this. If you have symptoms to warrant it, it may be appropriate to search for polyps or lumps in the rectum. More important, since the rectum (unlike the vagina) does not end in an impassable cul-de-sac some 11 cm. inside your body, this gives an opportunity to reach further inside. If it is important for the doctor to extend a sensitive finger around the back of the uterus, this may only be done via the rectum.

## BREAST EXAMINATION

As well as the bi-manual examination, your breasts will be examined. Some doctors prefer to do the internal examination before looking at breasts while some do it the other way round. If you have a strong preference one way or other, mention this to your doctor and negotiate a mutual agreement. The doctor will be looking for any signs that might indicate infection or tumours. You will be asked to strip off the top half of your clothes and to stand facing the doctor. You should then be instructed to raise your arms above your head and to turn from side to side, to allow the doctor to look at your breasts from all angles. Next, you should place your hands on your hips and press inwards, and then clasp your hands in front of you, tightly and quickly. Lumps may be too small to be felt, but can often show up with a tell-tale puckering of the skin over the affected area during these procedures. The doctor will examine the nipples and then press the flats of his or her fingers all over your breasts and into the armpit, searching for lumps. This examination is often done best twice – once standing and once lying down, as some lumps will only become apparent in one position.

If your doctor finds a lump that needs further investigation, there are several options. If it is highly likely that the growth is nothing more sinister than a cyst, a needle biopsy can be done on the spot, or you could be sent to an out-patient department for the procedure. The needle of a syringe is pushed into the lump and the lump is 'aspirated' – fluid is drawn out. If fluid *does* emerge, this is confirmation that the lump was no more than a cyst, and nothing more needs to be done. If the lump proves to be solid, you may be asked to go into hospital for a further test in which a section of the growth, or the whole growth, is excised and examined. The chances are that it will be benign rather than malignant, and the experience will leave no more than a slight and fading mark on your breast. It is worth noting that even malignant tumours can now often be treated 'conservatively' – that is, that the minimum of surgery may be done. Instead of removing the whole breast, in a mastectomy, frequently all that is necessary is for the tumour itself to be excised in a 'lumpectomy'. Considering the importance we place on our breasts, women who are told they should accept the mutilating surgery of a mastectomy might like to insist on proper discussion of alternatives and a second opinion.

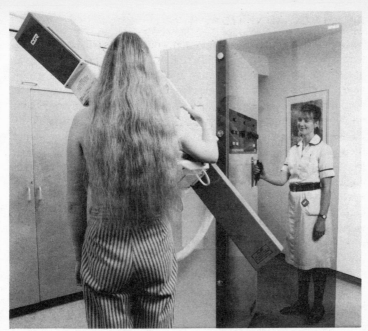

Two plastic sheets compress the woman's breast in preparation for an X-ray
mammography

If the doctor is unsure of the nature of any lump in your breast, or
unsure whether there might be lumps, you may be sent for a mammography. This is a special low-dose X-ray of the breasts themselves,
rather than the chest. The Fowler report on breast screening has
recommended that £50 million be made available for a national
breast-screening programme to be offered from regional centres to *all*
women aged between fifty and sixty. Women under fifty will need
their doctor's referral for such an examination. Many doctors are
happy to send their patients for a routine mammographic screening
if they fall within one of the risk groups.

Mammography can be a bit alarming and uncomfortable, although
it is not painful. Each breast is in turn pressed between two plates
and X-rayed. Any lump will show up, and an experienced clinician
can usually make a diagnosis or decide whether surgical examination
will then be needed. You might also be offered ultrasound or thermography. The first is more helpful in combination with mammography

rather than on its own. Thermography takes a 'heat' photograph of your body, and cancerous areas show up as being hotter than surrounding tissue. However, this technique is considered less effective today than mammography.

## SELF-EXAMINATION

The embarrassment that most of us feel when having an intimate examination comes from a confusing mixture of fear and expectations. In a society that makes nakedness taboo, being without clothes can make you feel extremely vulnerable. We normally only trust our unclothed bodies to the select few with whom we have very special emotional relationships – parents, children and lovers. Stripping off in front of a stranger puts an uncomfortable context on the act – does this sharing of intimate secrets make them intimate with us? That the examination *is* often in a sexual context, as part of a consultation that directly or indirectly touches on our sexual lives, makes the doctor/patient relationship all that more touchy and difficult. Since the doctor is looking for symptoms and problems – in other words, making a judgement on your body about whether everything is 'right' and nothing is 'wrong' – we can easily imagine that other judgements are being made. Are we 'clean' enough? Is our body unpleasant, unattractive, unusual? Is our sexuality or our sexual behaviour unacceptable, sinful, deviant or excessive? Are we 'up to scratch'?

Alternatively, we may often feel apologetic, because we see the areas that the doctor examines as his or her property, not our own. Our reproductive organs are medical territory, and knowledge about these parts is specialized and for the professionals alone. Thus, we are uneasy and apologetic because it is as if this area belongs to the doctors and we have misused it.

You have no need to feel like this. Your body belongs to *you* – it is not on loan from anyone else, however much more they know about its workings than you. And that knowledge is not the exclusive preserve of any professional. You have as much right to information as anyone else, and *more* right to use it to decide what to do about your own body.

For this reason, learning how to examine and get to know your own body is important. The more you are familiar with yourself, the more in control you can be about what is to happen, both in everyday circumstances and in the case of problems. Since any of the conditions that can harm, disable and even kill us develop slowly over a time, *we* – not our doctors – are often in the best position to 'whistle-blow'. 90 per cent of breast lumps are initially detected by the woman herself – although this fact may be more a measure of the lack of medical screening than our alertness! Some complaints are silent until a late stage, but many make themselves felt in visible changes or by making us experience pain, tiredness or depression. The more we know how our bodies look and feel in *good* health, the better our chances of picking up the subtle changes in the slide through less good to bad health. A change can be missed by a doctor, who is not as familiar as you could be with how you look and feel at your best. Needless to say, the earlier a problem is detected and treated, the better your chances of cure and recovery.

Self-examination should become a part of your routine – as much so as checking finger- and toe-nails for chips and growth. The basic bits of equipment you need to do this are:

- A private and comfortable place.
- A good source of light.
- A mirror.

It is also an excellent idea to get a speculum of your own. Like thermometers, these are not instruments only available to doctors, and are perfectly safe in your hands. Just as with a thermometer, you need to have a bit of common sense and care in using one. You do not need to use surgical gloves when examining yourself, but clean hands are a must.

The best time to examine yourself is in the week following your period – if you have passed the menopause, choose a time to suit yourself and try to repeat at monthly intervals after that. Set aside an uninterrupted half hour when you will not be called away and can relax. Make sure you are warm. You could, for instance, do this just after having a bath or shower. If you are worried about a discharge, of course, you will not want to remove evidence beforehand.

## BREAST SELF-EXAMINATION

Strip off and stand facing a mirror large enough to give you a full view of your breasts. Look at the nipples. Are they both around the same height? Is either nipple withdrawn – unless, that is, you have always had indrawing nipples? Is there a discharge from either nipple?

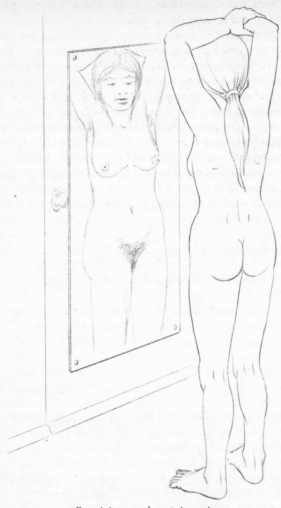

Examining your breasts in a mirror

You could squeeze them *gently* to check this. Are there any rashes, cracks or irritations? Now, raise your arms and look at your breasts. Can you see any dimpled or puckered areas when you move? Are any veins standing out more than they usually do? Put hands on hips and press inwards. Any sign of dimples or puckering? Clasp your hands in front and squeeze them together firmly, looking again for any changes in the surface of your breasts.

For the next stage, lie down on a firm surface. You may find it convenient to spread out on a towel or blanket on the floor. Place a folded towel under your left shoulder-blade to raise your body slightly. Raise your left hand and tuck it behind your head. With the right hand, you will now start feeling the breast to check its texture. There are two important points here. Firstly, use the *flats* of your fingers to do this, not your fingertips. Poking downwards with sensitive finger-tips will make you aware of every little duct and nodule, and give you the impression that your breasts are like a sack-full of ballbearings! By using the flats, you are able to press less harshly and to extend the sensitive 'sensor' area to give a better picture of whether there are any lumps that could cause alarm. Secondly, you may find it helpful to soap your hand and breast or to use a body lotion or cream. The sliding sensation gives you a better chance of feeling any bumps. If you can't use moisture or cream, spread a silk scarf over your breast, or slip a sheer nylon stocking or leg of a pair of tights over your hand. Again, this allows your fingers to slide over your body and become more sensitive.

Start above the breast, just below the collar-bone. Move your hand in a circle around the nipple, feeling or 'palpating' the breast. When you get back to your starting-point, move inwards the width of your fingers and continue until you end up at the nipple. Alternatively, you could mentally divide your breast up into sections that corres-pond to a clock face. Starting at twelve o'clock, move inwards until you have felt that section and then go to one o'clock and move inwards again, continuing round and in until the whole breast has been examined. According to some evidence, 45 per cent of breast cancers appear first in the outside, upper part, so be particularly careful to feel this area. However, note that this is also the most innocently lumpy area and that both malignant and benign tumours do arise anywhere in the breast. Finally, palpate up from the breast into the armpit.

You are likely to find that your breasts are *not* uniform in either appearance or feel. We all have networks of veins and stria – stretch-marks that appear as silvery or red lines just below the skin surface. Most women find that one breast is larger than the other, and nipples are unlikely to hang *exactly* equal. It is common to feel rubbery areas or notice what appear to be gritty deposits or strings of tiny bumps.

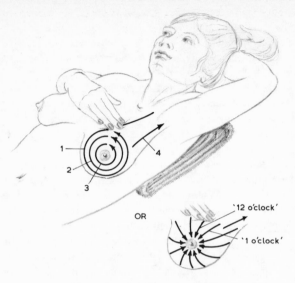

'12 o'clock'

OR

'1 o'clock'

Two sequences of breast palpitation

Regular self-examination will allow you to work out which of these are just part of normal development, as they recede and come back over a period – or need further tests if they stay the same or enlarge. Having examined one breast, shift the towel to the other shoulder-blade and repeat the exercise with the other breast.

## INTERNAL SELF-EXAMINATION

While lying down, go on to examine your vulva. You will need a mirror and a good light source for this. Prop yourself up on pillows or cushions, or lean back against a sofa arm (or the arm of a companion!), so you can see your vulva area clearly in the mirror without straining your neck or stomach muscles. You may need to prop up the mirror to leave both your hands free. Alternatively, crouch, squat or stand over your mirror. You could, for instance, place it on a low stool and straddle over it. Unless you have a specific infection, the vulva and the vagina are perfectly clean areas. The fluids that keep them moist also keep them healthy, and these secretions are in no way unhygienic. However, since the area is fragile, you need to be

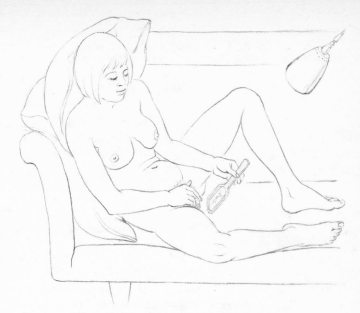

Self-examination of the vulva with the aid of a mirror

careful about not taking contamination *into* it. Before examining yourself, do make sure your hands are clean and your nails are smooth, so that there is no risk of your snagging them on the delicate tissue inside you. Remove any rings with sharp edges. If you have any open wounds on the fingers you intend introducing inside yourself, either get hold of a sterile surgical glove to wear or wait until the wound is healed – or use another finger.

Bend your knees and let them separate. Leave your feet flat on the floor or bed, or prop them up over the arms of a sofa or another pillow. With one or both hands, part your labia and have a look at them. Note the colour and texture, and see if there are any areas of roughness or redness, or any obvious sores. Look for the natural sebaceous glands, which may show as white bumps, and note the relative moistness or dryness of the inner lips or labia minora. Look for your clitoris, probably hidden by the prepuce or fold of skin formed by the front of the labia minora. The clitoris will probably show as a pink nub, surrounded by its darker hood. Working backwards (or, lying on your back, downwards) you can find the urethra or waste-water opening by parting the inner lips. Below that is the entrance to the vagina.

The vaginal opening is often shown as a gaping hole in illustrations. As you will find, it is actually held closed and flattened by the pressure of the closed legs, by the protection of the labia and by the tissue and muscle that surround it. The vagina only gapes open when the lips are parted and you introduce something into it. However, unless you are tense and clamp these muscles firmly shut, the tube of the vagina is enormously flexible. It will stretch easily to take several fingers, as it would for a tampon or a penis. Remember, as you look at and examine the vagina, that sometime in your life it may have to stretch to allow up to eight pounds of baby to emerge! If the vagina can do *that*, it can certainly accommodate fingers, tampons and penises! There is no such thing as a vagina that is too small for examination, internal sanitary protection or love-making.

If you do find yourself a bit dry, use some help to make the next part of the examination easier. A water-soluble (*not* a petroleum-based) cream or jelly is best – some KY Jelly, Durex lubricating jelly or Senselle. Or, if you use spermicidal cream as a method of contraception, try a blob of that. Otherwise, moisten your hand with water and a very small amount of *mild* soap.

Slide a finger inside the vagina. You may feel, and be able to see, some tags of tissue around the entrance, or you may find a ring of tissue just inside. This will be your hymen or maidenhead and should not be mistaken for suspicious lumps. Not every woman has a noticeable hymen. In some, it is firm and noticeable until you have penetrative sex, when it will either stretch or be broken. Indeed, the ring can remain intact until the vagina stretches for childbirth. In others, it is hardly present or is stretched or broken long before sexual intercourse.

The vagina itself may feel moist and the walls quite 'grainy'. Imagine what a silk stocking looks and feels like. When stretched over your leg, it is sheer and smooth, but when removed it may fall into folds and feel bumpy and irregular. Your relaxed vagina has deep folds running along its length, and a roughened texture.

Your longest finger, usually the second finger, may be able to reach right to the end of your vagina. Pressing down against the posterior (back or lower) wall, slide your finger inside as far as you can. You may be able to feel the vaginal vault – a cul-de-sac or dead-end some 7 to 10 cm. inside yourself. If you do this, but slide the finger, pressing it *upwards* against the front or upper wall, you will feel an obstruction or lump jutting out into the vagina at right angles to it, after some 6 to 8 cm. This is your cervix. By exploring the cervix with the tip of your finger you may find it resembles the end of your nose – firm, smooth and with a dimple in the middle. This dimple is the cervical os, the channel leading into the womb. You will find that you can move the cervix by gently pulling at it – and this, in turn, will make your uterus shift slightly. You may feel some deep sensations, but should feel no pain. Any pressing on the walls of the vagina could also result in referred sensations to other organs. If your bladder is full, pressing on the upper wall will make you want to pass water, and a full bowel could be felt through the lower wall. By this exploration, you will become aware of the startling thinness, though sturdiness, of the walls of these parts of your body. If you have had a hysterectomy involving the removal of your cervix, you will find that the protruding lump is missing. Instead, your vagina is a closed cul-de-sac, with the area that was once interrupted by the cervix sealed with stitches. You may be able to feel scar tissue there. More usually, the area will feel like the rest of the vagina.

When you have become adept at self-examination, you might like to do your own bi-manual. While the finger of one hand is in your vagina, use the flat of the fingers on your other hand to gently press down on your lower belly, and see what you can feel between them. Do *not* press too hard, and also be prepared for the sensations to be a bit confusing and puzzling. It takes time and experience for a doctor to be able to interpret these sensations meaningfully and you are unlikely to be able to do so in a short time. But it can be fascinating to try!

Letting your fingers do the walking has one disadvantage. Finger-ends are so very sensitive that they can give us an exaggerated idea of what is there between our legs or inside us. Using the mirror to check your impressions while examining the vulva and entrance to the vagina is thus vital. It is also a good idea to match what you have *felt* with what you could *see*, by using a speculum.

## THE SPECULUM

It is very easy to imagine that a speculum is a 'doctor's-only' piece of equipment. You never see them on sale, and some chemists will sell them only on special request, and then only to the woman who can produce a supporting letter from a doctor! The argument is that, unless properly trained, you could do yourself some damage while inserting one of these devices. Yet chemists do not demand letters from dentists before selling you toothpicks – sharp instruments that can puncture gums! And who asks for proof that you already know what you are doing before selling you tampons? A speculum is no more dangerous or difficult to use than these. If your local chemist cannot help, a stockist who will supply by mail order is suggested at the end of the book.

The main provisos to keep in mind when using a speculum are:

1. Just as you are unlikely to feel happy about sharing a toothbrush with even your nearest and dearest, keep your speculum strictly for your own use.
2. Wash it carefully before and after use.
3. Insert it gently, slowly and carefully, so as not to scrape the delicate walls of the vagina.

When using the speculum, hold it hinge-side up and put some lubricating cream on the end. Holding it in one hand, as you would a tampon, part your vaginal lips with the other hand and introduce the end of the speculum inside the entrance to the vagina, and slide it inside you. When the 'bills' have been passed inside you and the hinge end has come up flat against your vulva, carefully operate the hinge and its ratchet. When it is in place and open, you will not have to hold the speculum to keep it inside you, although if you do move around or stand up, it *is* likely to fall or be pushed out. Now, hold your mirror and shine the light source inside yourself. You may find the most efficient way of doing this is to shine the light *on* the mirror and to direct the reflected light on to yourself. Looking through the circular end of the speculum, you will be able to see down the entire length of the vagina to the cervix. Note the colour and state of the vaginal walls, and the colour and appearance of the cervix. When you do want to remove the speculum, remember to do so with it still in the open position, otherwise you may nip yourself.

Self-examination should never be seen as a replacement for regular professional medical checks. It cannot be too strongly emphasized that pre-cancerous changes of the vagina and cervix, and often of the uterus, cannot be seen with the naked eye, but can be detected with a proper smear test long before obvious symptoms make themselves felt. At that stage, quick, easy and foolproof treatment is possible. If

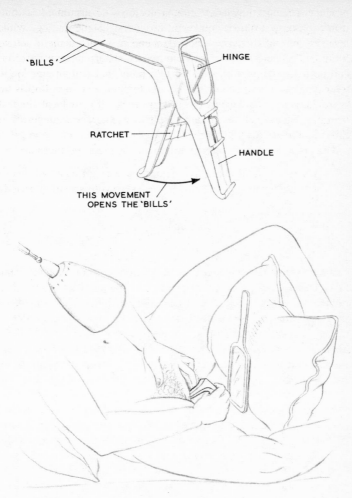

A plastic speculum and self-examination with the aid of the speculum, a mirror and reflected light

left until you can feel or see problems, the situation is far more difficult. But at *whatever* stage, the earlier the better. Nothing, be it cancer or thrush, goes away by being ignored.

However, this does not mean that self-help checks are a waste of time. Cancer is only the tip of the iceberg. There are a host of troublesome conditions that *could* arise, that you would be able to spot and have put right if you kept a running check on yourself. Most of the time these can only be noticed when you see a *change* – a slow and subtle alteration from what is normal for *you*. Even the most skilled doctor can miss this, for he or she *cannot* be as familiar with the everyday and normal state of your body as you *could* be if you looked!

Some doctors might feel challenged and resentful when faced by a patient who displays this sort of knowledge and control. You might find yourself labelled a 'know-it-all', an hysteric or a trouble-maker. You may find your remarks or questions dismissed with, 'What do you want to know that for?' or 'Why don't *you* let me do *my* job?' Such reactions, however, are becoming rarer.

The doctors' governing body – the British Medical Association – has declared itself fully in favour of women using any device or action they find acceptable and safe to learn about their bodies. They have specifically welcomed women using speculums to examine themselves and do not think it necessary for you to have training from doctors before doing so: you can learn perfectly well from a good magazine article or book such as this. Most doctors welcome the idea of health care being a *shared* responsibility between them and their patients. It is far easier for doctors to do their job when patients are willing to ask questions. Communication is far easier if patients have some knowledge and experience on which to base their questions and discussion.

Doctors operate under several handicaps when faced by a woman with a troublesome symptom or condition. If male, however sympathetic and experienced, he will be unable to *empathize* or totally share in a related experience. It is very difficult to understand how it feels to have a pain in the breast or located around the pelvic organs if you have no breasts or pelvic organs! Both you and the doctor may then be further handicapped if he has been taught that women tend to exaggerate, are prone to be weak and hysterical, or that such pains are a natural and acceptable part of the female condition. Even given a female doctor or nurse, or a professional of either sex who is prepared to listen and to accept that if you *say* you have a pain, pain exists, it is still difficult to interpret one person's assessment of discomfort. Just as a given amount of menstrual blood may be seen as excessive, normal or light by different women, so pain and discomfort is something that can be tolerated or not by different people.

The most important contribution you can make to overcoming your doctor's difficulties, then, is an accurate and unexaggerated reporting of symptoms and impressions, and an unshakeable faith in your ability to *know* your body and be right when you say something is wrong. Certainty and conviction are catching, as is lack of confidence. Some doctors are unenthusiastic about screening, for economic reasons. It has been suggested that cytology screening for young people is a waste of time and money since true cancer is extremely rare in the under thirty-fives and abnormalities, when they are found, frequently revert to normal without treatment – all that screening achieves is needless anxiety on the part of the woman and a screening service so bogged down with unnecessary tests that it cannot extend a service to the people who really need it.

What this argument ignores is the fact that the reason women die in their fifties and sixties from reproductive cancers is mostly because they do not go for testing: and they do not go for testing because the procedure is unfamiliar and thus frightening. If we could make such tests a routine part of our lives from a very early age, we would be happily part of the system by the time it really becomes essential. The benefits from having a smear test at thirty-five may not be apparent for ten to fifteen years, while the benefit of having one at forty can be immediate. But if you do not start until you are fifty, the chances are you may not start at all.

# CHAPTER 4

# *Self-Help*

It is easy to assume that our state of health is something that happens *to* us. We tend to be fatalistic about fitness or illness, considering those with energy to spare are 'lucky' and talking about 'falling ill', as if neither had anything to do with our behaviour or lifestyle. We eat unhealthy diets and indulge in all sorts of unhealthy practices, thinking that 'If this was really so bad, THEY would ban it.' When illness arrives and doctors cannot provide an immediate and magic cure, we blame them. It's their responsibility to look after us, so a failure is their fault.

These beliefs, while understandable, are inaccurate and unhelpful. There is plenty of evidence linking disease and ill health to the environment in which we live and work, and to our own actions.

Well Woman care is based on our accepting and taking responsibility for ourselves. This should *not* mean that if illness strikes we should in any way feel guilty. Nor should it mean that we must assume that all health care should come from ourselves and that doctors are irrelevant. The only danger in Well Woman care is when we use it to avoid or delay seeking necessary professional attention, and when we blame ourselves for illness that *is* beyond our control. So, what are the factors that contribute to our well-being or lack of it, and how can we influence them? Our eating, smoking and drinking habits, our physical fitness, our sexual behaviour – all contribute to whether or not we develop certain difficulties. All of these are elements that we *can* change and adapt to suit both our own taste and our own health.

Certain cancers are a perfect example of this. You cannot *catch* cancer. What you can do is increase the possibility of certain cells in your body undergoing the changes that lead to cancer. It would appear that some people inherit a tendency to certain cancers – breast cancer, for instance. But your environment has far more of an effect on your chances of developing disease than your genes. Frequently, it is not that you inherit a genetic risk from your parents and their generation, but that you copy their way of living, and this puts you at risk.

## SEX AND CANCER

There is a well-established link between our sexual history and certain cancers of the reproductive organs. Cancer of the cervix occurs least among nuns and homosexual women, and most among women with multiple sexual partners. The link, however, is not just an easy question of saying that sexual promiscuity leads to cancer. After all, what is a definition of promiscuity? Having had sex with two men in a lifetime? Two men in a night? As one sexual expert has pointed out, a promiscuous person tends to be defined as someone who has slept with one more person than the person making the definition! Furthermore, celibate women are more likely to suffer tumours of the breast than their sexually active sisters.

The sexual link with cancer is complex. The cells on the surface of the cervix can be affected by an outside agent and become more prone to go through the changes that lead to cancer. Women who start their sex lives quite early are more likely to suffer these changes – probably because the cells at this stage are not yet fully mature and are liable to be affected. The causative agent is thought to be present in the man's sperm. Some men are more likely to have this effect than others, and men who have been infected by STDs – especially genital warts – are most likely of all. Women who themselves become infected by STDs are more likely to go on to develop cancer of the cervix, especially those who are infected by the genital wart virus or the herpes virus. Early pregnancy is also linked with cervical cancer, even in a woman who has only had one sexual partner and no STDs. It has even been suggested that men in some occupations, especially those who come into contact with certain chemicals, can prove risky. However, researchers are not certain of the link and suggest it may have more to do with basic hygiene and the fact that men in some of the suggested high-risk occupations are more likely to have opportunities for promiscuous sexual behaviour, rather than a carcinogenic property of the chemicals concerned.

However, the sexual links are no reason for you to feel that being offered or asking for a smear test is a slur on your character or a comment on your relationship. There is no stigma attached to the test and having it done will *not* brand you as being promiscuous.

As already mentioned, breast cancer has a strong tendency to run in families. If your sister or mother has had breast cancer, you are two or three times more likely to develop a malignant tumour too – particularly if they were pre-menopausal at the time or if the tumours occurred in both breasts. Women who start their periods early (before the age of twelve) or enter menopause late (after fifty) – the two also seem to go together and, again, go in families – are at greater risk than women who have a shorter time of being fertile. Another risk-factor is delaying pregnancy until your thirties, or never having children. So it is not so much your *sex* life as your *reproductive* life that is important, although the two tend to go together. It appears that subjecting your breasts to the hormonal levels of an ovulating woman for a long time is harmful. This is probably why some studies suggest that a diet high in fats increases your risks of developing breast cancer – dairy fats can increase the amount of the hormone prolactin found in your system. One in seventeen women in the UK will be diagnosed as having breast cancer. The rate in Japan is one in forty – the Japanese diet is very low in dairy products and other saturated fats, and this is thought to be a significant factor. Some studies suggest that being on the Pill has some adverse effect, although other reports do not confirm these findings.

## SMOKING

As well as increasing your chances of developing lung cancer, cigarette smoking can increase your risk of developing cancer of the cervix. Cigarette smokers are also more likely to suffer from pre-menstrual syndrome and to go into menopause around two years earlier than they would otherwise have done. To add insult to injury, smokers also suffer from far more facial wrinkles than do non-smokers. So much so, that some doctors call it 'smokers' face' and sometimes can tell if you smoke just by looking at you. If you continue smoking after the menopause, you are also more likely than a non-smoker to suffer a distressing condition called osteoporosis. This is when the calcium leaches from your bones, leaving them brittle and at risk of breaking.

Osteoporosis tends to start after menopause when the body scales down its production of oestrogen. Post-menopausal women are ten times as likely to suffer from fractures of the hip, thigh and wrist than men of the same age. Bone-loss is most rapid in the first five years after menopause and, after ten to fifteen years, as much as one third of skeletal mass could have been lost. At this stage, not only will the spine slowly impact, making you shorter, but it will also bend, giving you the characteristic 'Dowager's Hump'. It has been estimated that the cost to the NHS of treating fractures of the wrist alone amounts to some £100 million a year.

## DRINKING

Although the Bible enjoins, 'Use a little wine for thy stomach's sake and thine often infirmities', and *moderate* wine consumption may be good for the heart and circulation, there does seem to be a link between even moderate drinking and breast cancer. Your chances of damaging both your body and your social life are definitely increased by even an apparently low level of regular drinking. The safe limit suggested by some experts for women is no more than thirteen units a week. A unit is half a pint of beer, a single pub measure of spirits (home measures tend to be larger!) or a standard-sized glass of wine, sherry or fortified wine. Men can drink a little more than the average woman due to their greater size and a slightly different body composition. The general rule is that men can drink two or three pints or their equivalent, two or three times a week, and that women can have two or three units two or three times a week to keep within a fairly safe limit. Any more, and the first thing you will notice to suffer is your waistline. However, it has also been suggested that as little as three glasses of wine a week increases your risks of developing breast cancer by 50 per cent.

## OBESITY

Being overweight also has its attendant health problems. Extra weight puts a strain on the heart, increasing your risk of heart disease and raising your blood-pressure. The added burden on your joints can encourage wear and tear and lead to arthritis. Extra weight may also affect the hormone system, leading to difficulties in achieving a wanted pregnancy. We tend to think of weight as only being a cosmetic problem, and some women quite rightly react against the demand that we always be slim, attractive and sexually available, and assert that fat is beautiful too. That may be, but in choosing to be overweight, you should at least recognize that you are also choosing to risk a wide range of health problems. If being overweight is not your choice, but you find it difficult to shed extra pounds, perhaps the goal of a lifetime's health is a better and more practical one to strive after than being beautiful. Not all of us can achieve the latter, but we can *all* make great strides towards the former.

Pursuing your ideal weight through yet one more magic, easy diet is unlikely to help you very much. Diets often do not address the basic problem, which is that too many of us habitually eat too much fat and refined sugar and not enough fresh produce and fibre, and very few of us exercise our bodies as much as they were intended to be. You will spend your life in an endless battle with fat if you veer between stringent low-calorie regimens and a 'normal' pattern of treats in the form of cakes and chips, and see getting hot, sweaty and keeping fit as unfeminine, too much like hard work or boring. The word 'diet' should not mean a punishing, short-term regimen. It should refer to your everyday, lifetime pattern of eating. As such, it can contain the safe and sensible amounts of good food, shed large quantities of dangerous and unhealthy stuff, and *still* be exciting, varied and enjoyable. Similarly, as many people have found, taking up a sport can be fun as well as having quite a staggering effect on your weight and well-being.

## KEEPING FIT

There are considerable barriers between most women and exercise. Many of us have unpleasant memories of school sports and find the idea of running around getting hot and sweaty very off-putting. Any benefits from sport can be slow in coming, while the discomfort and inconvenience is immediate! We may not have suitable clothing, suitable footwear or a suitable hairstyle for exercising, and may be reluctant to 'make a fool of ourselves' in front of other people. We may have justified fears of going out on our own – lone women joggers and walkers can be a target for harassment ranging from unpleasant remarks to physical assault. Our families can be less than helpful, either being resentful of time spent on our 'selfish' pursuits away from them, or feeling intimidated or jealous of the new 'athletic' you. Children, particularly, can be mortified and embarrassed at Mum getting up to such undignified antics.

## STRESS

Of course, worrying about our health can in itself lead to problems. Perhaps the biggest killer and contributor to ill health in our society is *stress*. Stress is a necessary and helpful state in certain circumstances and in small doses. It is a state of mind and body in which you are 'keyed-up' to act quickly and efficiently. It was stress that enabled our ancestors to tread lightly when walking near a dangerous predator, or while stalking their supper. It is stress that enables you to be ready and to react to a child in danger, or to plan and carry out a difficult job at home or work. Stress makes you a better driver and a safer pedestrian. In a stressed state, our adrenal glands secrete quantities of the hormone adrenalin into the bloodstream, to make the heart beat faster and the muscles react more quickly. Problems arise, however, when this happens more often than we need. If we do not have to call on these extra reserves and burn off the energy we have on tap, the constant up and down of our physical state becomes harmful. High blood-pressure, heart disease and stomach ulcers can be the physical results. We may show our tension in eating too much or too little, or in smoking or drinking – all of which, in turn, take a physical toll.

## ENVIRONMENTAL HAZARDS

We cannot exclude our living and working conditions from the factors that affect health. Whether we work in or outside the home, we are exposed to physical, chemical, biological and psychological influences which may be hazardous to varying degrees. *Physical hazards* can come from noise, vibration, dangerous machinery, lighting, temperature, radiation, or from the effects of lifting heavy weights, being too long on your feet or from badly designed seating. *Chemical hazards* can come from dust, fumes, gases and vapours, chemical liquids and solids. *Biological hazards* can come from germs from dirty conditions or from contact with infected material in hospitals or laboratories. *Psychological hazards* can come from stress, boredom, overwork or harassment.

Women are also at risk of suffering violence in the home, loneliness, poverty and crippling low self-esteem. These are even more prevalent among women who do not have full-time paid jobs or who are the main breadwinners in their family. All this may go some way towards explaining why cancers of many types, including those of the reproductive organs, and other illnesses, are more likely in women at the lower end of the social scale. Class relates to poverty, and the poorer you are the more difficult it is to pursue a healthy lifestyle. Not only can you not afford it, but the dice are loaded against your having the motivation to seize control over your life and your being able to stand up against the barriers that come between you and well-being.

Your ideal, then, is to be born into an upper-class family, with no history of cancer; to have a late menarche and early menopause; to delay starting your sexual life until your mid-twenties, or to use a condom at every sexual encounter before then. You should get pregnant at this time with the help of a non-promiscuous man who is certifiably free from STDs and preferably a virgin. You should both then remain faithful to each other, while remaining laid-back non-smokers who take only the occasional glass of wine with your low-fat diet, eaten between visits to your gym or squash court. Both of you should have professional jobs which do not bring you into contact with any hazardous material.

## WHAT YOU CAN DO

If the Good Lord has not obliged by placing you in such an ideal position, what can you do for yourself? Accidents of birth aside, you *can* use your awareness of your own body and your right to good health to arrange your lifestyle around a healthy existence. This does *not* mean using stringent diets or douches or feminine deodorants to achieve some advertising man's ideal of the Perfect Woman. Neither does it mean swallowing vitamin supplements. If you eat fresh food in the proper quantities, you should be getting all the vitamins and minerals you need (although there might be some specific exceptions – see later). And healthy eating and regular exercise are a lot more fun than many of us realize.

So, how can you arrange your life around good health? Firstly, accept the cliché that 'you are what you eat'. Eating patterns probably cause more problems to women than anything else, whether you are a single woman catering for yourself or a mother with a family. Most of us have some element of pressure that affects the way we buy, cook and serve our food. It can be economic – a tight budget often dictates what is on the shopping list. Or it may be lack of time, for the

woman with both an outside paid job and a home to run. The pref-
erences of the people who share our table also have a lot to do with
what is on offer. What is the point in cooking and serving what we
know is 'good' food if it only leads to whines, arguments and waste?
Whatever the pressure, the chances are that we will have found that
the easiest fare to offer has an excess of fat and sugar over the more
nutritious elements we really need. Many diets are low in fibre. A
high-fibre diet not only helps you avoid putting on weight, it protects
against bowel problems, including cancer.

If you want to increase your long-term chances of becoming and
staying healthy, you really *have* to opt for a healthy diet. This means
being sparing over the number of packaged foods you use – they use
large amounts of sugar, salt and fat – and becoming more generous
with fresh and high-fibre ingredients such as wholemeal bread and
pasta. It may mean spending more time on shopping and preparation,
to seek out the cheaper bargains in seasonal fruit and vegetables,
meat and fish, and to combine them into delicious meals. The questions to ask yourself if you are finding this hard are:

1. What about a contribution from the other people who are
going to eat this meal? Would it really be so unreasonable to ask
someone else to do part of the shopping or to take turns in being
responsible for it? And why not have a family 'cook-in' with all of
you swopping chat and news while sharing the preparation of the
meal?

2. If you think this takes too long, what are you saving time *for*? If
you feel too tired, might it not be because you're exhausted from the
effects of a poor diet and not enough exercise, than because making a
proper meal is really too much work?

Often we have a preference for fatty, sweet food because it has
become a habit, rather than because the alternative is actually less
palatable. Fresh flavours can seem bland at first after the thicker,
more cloying sensations of artificial flavours. If you can hold out
against the clamourings and the complaints of your own appetite
and those of your family, you are likely to find that 'better' food soon
becomes preferable, as well. You do not have to struggle to change
your situation on your own. Your doctor would like to help, knowing
the risks of being overweight and eating badly and knowing that help
now saves NHS money in the long run. Organizations such as Weight

Watchers and Slimming Magazine Clubs can give you valuable help and support. You will find their addresses listed later in the book.

Exercise can have a remarkable effect on your health and well-being. Some years ago, the media had a field day when the 'guru' of jogging, Jim Fixx, died in his mid-fifties of a heart attack while out running. What few of the stories mentioned was the fact that Fixx had an inherited heart condition, from which his father had died in *his* mid-forties. In effect, regular exercise had probably bought Fixx an extra ten productive, healthy and happy years of life.

The key to letting exercise do something for you is to begin slowly and to build up. Work out whether you need company and encouragement, or would be happier doing it on your own. If the first, join a class or group in your local leisure centre or elsewhere. There are very few places in the British Isles nowadays that are not within spitting distance of some sort of keep-fit class, and if you *are* the exception, start your own! Get together with a few friends or neighbours to exercise to a tape or record, or go jogging. You will find that not only do you begin to see some effect on your waistline and general sense of well-being after a few months, but that your social life may improve as well.

While looking at your food, you might next cast a critical eye on the other substances you take in. How much alcohol do you drink? If you are in the habit of consuming more than thirteen units a week, you are at risk. Cutting down makes sense, especially with the wide range of low-alcohol or alcohol-free drinks carried these days by every pub and eating place. If you find giving up a problem, there are specialized groups to turn to as well as your own doctor.

While a moderate level of drinking is unlikely to do you much harm, *any* level of cigarette smoking increases your risk of suffering lung cancer or cancer of the cervix. Furthermore, children of smokers have a higher risk of suffering bronchial and other illnesses. The dangers of passive smoking – of developing health problems from inhaling someone else's cigarette smoke – are beginning to be well documented. More and more workplaces and public areas are helping the majority who do not smoke to assert their right to clean lungs – and helping those who do smoke to give up – by banning smoking. Your doctor would only be too delighted to help you give up. There is a wide range of free, helpful leaflets and inexpensive books to give you support, as well as some excellent self-help groups. You can find these listed at the end of this book. If you would like to make your workplace a non-smoking area and your employer has not already taken this initiative, contact your union representative or the local Health and Safety Officer for advice. For safety reasons if no other, most employers should be delighted to agree.

Addiction to substances such as tranquillizers and other prescribed drugs, as well as illegal materials, can only be harmful. Again, most doctors are now aware of the professional mistakes that have been made in the past in over-prescribing or inappropriate prescribing, and would like to help. There are groups, leaflets and books suggested later on.

All of these problems can be tackled by you, but you do not have to struggle on your own. There is an enormous and extremely helpful range of publications – books, booklets and leaflets – to aid you, whether you want to change your eating habits, give up smoking or taking tranquillizers, or get fit. Even more helpful for many people is the widespread existence of support groups. These are sometimes run by professional counsellors and sometimes by people who have had a particular problem themselves. Whatever you want to give up, or encourage yourself to take up, you will find enthusiastic companions if you look for them. Isolation and the nagging feeling that your problem or difficulty in handling it is unique, are often your worst enemies in seeking an optimally healthy lifestyle. It can be liberating and remarkably effective to come out in the open where you can find others in the same situation, and together seek a solution. You may find something as simple and seemingly irrelevant as a mothers-and-toddlers playgroup or an evening class can help with weight problems! Many of our difficulties are increased by stress and loneliness, so anything that can relieve pressure and make us feel more relaxed and happy about ourselves can help.

## SELF-TREATMENT

As well as taking preventative steps to make it less likely that you will suffer ill health, there are some conditions you can treat on your own. In many cases, simple problems will respond as well or better to the sorts of measures you can apply yourself. Equally, the action you can take on your own will be the same as that suggested by a doctor. The common cold, for instance, will respond no more quickly to anything your doctor can give you. A few days of looking after yourself at home, dosing yourself with aspirin to relieve symptoms, good food to strengthen your body and its immune system, and warmth to make you feel better, are all you need. The doctor is only necessary to reassure you that a cold *is* what you have, and not something more serious. If you know the symptoms, you need only your own common sense.

Similarly, you certainly could *start* treatment for conditions such as cystitis, thrush and PMS on your own. In all cases, you can give a doctor valuable information if, when you become aware of an itch or discharge, a rash or a lump or pain, you can note its development and give him or her a proper and detailed description.

## THRUSH

Thrush often responds well to home-based methods of treatment. The key to fighting this yeast- or fungus-like condition is to restore the naturally acidic nature of your vaginal fluid. If you can do this, the environment in which candida moniliasis flourishes will disappear. At the first signs of the white, thick, yeasty-smelling discharge, or the itchy rash that often accompanies it, cut out as much sugar and yeast as possible from your diet. Resist the temptation to wash or bathe more often – moist heat only encourages candida. Instead, only wash in tepid water twice a day. Buy a tub of *live*, unsweetened, natural yoghurt – many supermarkets carry this now, and any health-food store would have some. Soak a tampon in it and then insert it into your vagina. If the yoghurt is very thick, dilute it first with a little warm water. You could also use a weak solution of vinegar or lemon juice: put a tablespoon of the acid in half a pint of warm water, soak a tampon in the solution and insert it into your vagina, leaving it for a few hours before changing tampons. You could also add vinegar or lemon juice to your bath water. When you bathe, lift your hips under the water while using your fingers to gently open your vagina, allowing the treated water to flow inside. If all this sounds a bit off, think about the fruit and vegetables we happily spread over ourselves in the form of coconut-oil soap, cocoa-butter shampoo and avocado moisturizing cream.

When treating yourself, do not forget to ask your sexual partner (if you have one) to take steps too. Men rarely suffer from thrush, but can harbour the fungus and pass it back to their partners if they, too, do not seek treatment. Using vinegar or lemon juice in the bath or washing water and dunking the male organ in live yoghurt can help!

Thrush is one of the few genital conditions that can be passed between homosexual women, so being gay is no protection against picking up this particular problem.

One-off attacks of thrush can be nipped in the bud thoroughly and successfully by treatment prescribed by your doctor. Anti-fungal creams, pessaries, powders and tablets can kill off the condition. However, recurrent and chronic cases often need non-medical remedies as well. If you are prone to developing thrush, the sooner you respond to an attack the easier it will be to divert it. The more you avoid the conditions that encourage thrush the better. So, avoid sugary food, frequent hot baths and tight, restricting clothing around the vagina. Although not always avoidable, pregnancy, the Pill and antibiotics can also encourage thrush.

## CYSTITIS

Cystitis is another condition that you *can* treat yourself. However, more care is needed than with thrush. Failing to contain thrush may mean you have to endure a longer and more uncomfortable bout of the condition but, however exhausting and unpleasant, it does no lasting damage. Our response to treatment is also individual and, while for some, prescribed treatment does the trick, others find over-the-counter, self-administered means are actually better. Cystitis, however, can cause havoc if allowed to travel from the bladder up into the kidneys. For this reason, self-treatment should only be used as an immediate response before seeking medical help. If it cures an attack, as it may, then well and good. If not, go for professional help.

At the *first* signs of an attack – a nagging desire to pass water that stays even after you have been to the lavatory, pain occurring on passing water, bloody or cloudy urine or an ache around the groin – drink plenty of water, at least a pint. Avoid acids, such as fruit juices, but add either bicarbonate of soda or barley water to the liquid or one of the new proprietary treatments available over the counter from your chemist. If you have high blood-pressure or suffer from heart problems, ask a doctor before using bicarbonate of soda in this way. Make yourself comfortable with some soothing hot-water bottles, and some pain-killers if you need them. Then, over the next three hours, try to drink *at least* another four pints of water – a half pint every twenty minutes. Every hour, add a teaspoon of bicarb to your half pint. Weak tea or coffee can help make all this fluid palatable, and the caffeine also encourages you to pass water quickly. However, some people find caffeine increases their discomfort – you will have to work out for yourself if this is true for you. Herbal teas can be a useful alternative, and several are particularly recommended as being helpful in cystitis cases – marshmallow, camomile, fennel and thyme. Some herbalists and healthfood stores sell a specific 'cystitis tea mix' using a combination of these. The more liquid you drink and the more you pass, the quicker the germs causing the cystitis will be flushed away, allowing your body to deal with the inflammation. If you follow this plan, most attacks of cystitis will be relieved after three hours. To prevent further attacks, remember to:

1. Always wipe from front to back after having a bowel movement. Carry some 'wet-wipe' tissues with you – the type usually used to clean babies – and use them to clean up thoroughly.

2. Make a habit of nipping to the bathroom just before and after making love. Sex on a full bladder can cause irritation, and flushing out the urethra after intercourse can usually drive out any harmful bacteria before they take hold.

3. Drink plenty of liquid, but avoid strong tea, coffee or alcohol.

4. Don't 'hang on' when you want to pass water – get to a loo as soon as possible.

5. Avoid tight clothing around your vulva, especially clothing made from artificial fibres.

6. Avoid bath oils and salts if these irritate you – and never use deodorants on the vulva.

If pain or discomfort lingers after this regimen, see a doctor for further help.


## PERIOD PROBLEMS

Many period problems respond to self-help remedies. You could obviously try to deal with period discomfort with self-administered painkillers. However, there are other even more effective responses. A bout of exercise – jogging, a keep-fit class, a game of squash – followed by a soothing hot bath can work wonders. We tend to have used period pain as an excuse to get out of games at school, and see exertion as something to avoid at this time in the month. A pity, since it can in fact help considerably. Extended exercise triggers the body to manufacture substances called endorphins, which are naturally occurring opiates. These kill pain and make you feel 'high' in perfect safety. Alternatively, use yoga or some other form of stress-releasing relaxation to help yourself unwind. Diet can play an important part in helping your body adjust to the normal ups and downs of the menstrual cycle. Herbal teas are said by some women to help ease period pain. They can also cut down on the 'bloated' feeling caused by fluid retention at this time, without giving you the nausea and irritation you may suffer from too much caffeine in coffee or ordinary tea. Herbal teas made from raspberry leaf, fennel, winter savory or pennyroyal are particularly recommended. Period pains also respond well to massage, and to orgasm – whether brought on by self-pleasuring or by contact with a sexual partner.

## PRE-MENSTRUAL SYNDROME (PMS)

Diet would also seem to have a large part in both creating and solving many of the problems relating to PMS. Sufferers often report cravings for sweet foods as part of their symptoms, yet a diet low in fat and sweet foods but high in fresh, raw and wholesome food is reported to help or relieve symptoms. On the whole, the taking of vitamin supplements is not proven to be of any value. The vitamins and minerals necessary to the human body are present in ample amounts in a healthy diet. You would obviously be deficient if you existed on over-cooked, packaged junk food, and in such cases a handful of pills every day *might* redress the balance. You would find it cheaper, far more pleasant and better for your waistline to eat well in the first place!

There is, however, a well-documented exception in that women suffering from PMS can respond dramatically to extra vitamin B6 or pyridoxine. This is available from chemists or healthfood stores without prescription, usually in tablets of 20 or 50 mg. It is suggested that you start on a dosage of 1 × 20 mg. twice a day – morning and night, after food. Start taking the tablets three days before you normally expect symptoms to begin, and continue until two days into your period. If this does not work, increase the dose the following month, up to a maximum of 75 mg. twice a day. Pyridoxine is safe, but it has been reported that a massive overdose can lead to loss of feeling in hands and feet – so if 150 mg. a day does not give relief, have a chat to your doctor. The vitamin B6 is naturally present in wheatgerm and bran, offal such as liver, kidney or hearts, egg yolks, black molasses, nuts, cabbage, tomatoes, avocado pears, bananas and brewers yeast. It would not be too hard to include all these in an interesting shopping list! Another dietary addition that has been found to help with PMS is gamma-linolenic acid (GLA), which is found in Evening Primrose oil. This, too, can be bought over the counter from a chemist or healthfood store under the name of Efamol, as well as being found in wheatgerm, sunflower and safflower seed oil, nuts and seeds. A suggested regimen is 2 or 3 × 500 mg. capsules, twice a day after food. It is also advisable to take extra vitamin C or ascorbic acid at the same time – 600 mg. daily – or to take Efamite, which contains vitamin C, B6 and zinc. Both zinc and magnesium deficiencies have been suggested as being significant in PMS. Both are found in sufficient quantities in red meat and unmilled cereals. Magnesium is also found in offal and green vegetables.

Unlike thrush and cystitis, the changes that occur around our menstrual cycle are not always necessarily to be thought of as problems in need of a cure. Much of our difficulty with periods can be traced to an attitude. If you have been brought up to see them as 'the curse', 'women's problems', messy, inconvenient and, above all, embarrassing and not to be discussed in male or polite society, then it is easy to find them problematical. Any discomfort will be magnified by feelings of disgust or resentment. If, however, you learn to appreciate and accept monthly changes as a natural and unremarkable *positive* aspect, and openly talk about and share your emotions and impressions with other people, you may find a difference in how you *feel*. This approach then means that if you *do* decide the pain or discomfort *is* unacceptable, you will not be put off by anyone trying to insist that you are being unreasonable.

Our main difficulty as women has been that, for centuries, those who look after our health – the medical profession – and those who present a picture of our society – our artists and writers – have primarily been men. The 'norm' has been the male – a static human being, one whose body and emotions have basically remained the same from one day to the next, except for one short major upheaval during puberty.

Women, although they represent 52 per cent of this planet's human beings, are still seen as not different, but substandard – 'men with a problem'. Between menarche and menopause, our bodies ride a switchback from one month to the next. Coping with this is like the difference between trying to stand in three feet of river water or three feet of sea water. If you apply the same rules – stand upright and steady – to the second as you do to the first, you are liable to be knocked off your feet and splashed. The key, then, is to adapt and learn to sway back and forth, enjoying the change of scenery and the pleasant rocking motion this gives you. If the sea gets rough, shout for a lifebelt, but don't let anyone tell you that the water is supposed to be calm and all those waves are in your imagination, or that you should accept being ducked and battered; neither is true.

## MENOPAUSE

Menopause, although a natural progression, can give rise to intolerable discomfort and genuine problems. Menopause describes the stopping of periods, an event that happens in the mid-forties to -fifties, although it does happen earlier or later in some women. Just as the menarche is only one aspect of puberty, so the menopause is only one part of the climacteric. This transition – from being a woman who can become pregnant to a woman who cannot – occurs over a five- to ten-year span. Most women spend a third of their lifetime as post-menopausal and this group represents 16 per cent of the population.

During the climacteric, oestrogen production in the ovaries decreases gradually. Periods become erratic and as many as 80 per cent of women develop oestrogen-deficient symptoms of varying intensity. 35 per cent of women find these bad enough for them to seek help from a doctor while the rest try to cope on their own.

Hot flushes, mood changes, depression, difficulty in sleeping, vaginal dryness, loss of sexual interest, tiredness, cystitis, bowel difficulties – all may crop up. Later on, you may well suffer from osteoporosis, having brittle bones due to calcium deficiency.

Diet, exercise and a commitment to accepting and looking after yourself, as well as other people, can make an enormous difference to how you weather the menopause. So too can a long, hard look at how much you value yourself. Post-menopausal women do have a dietary dilemma. Sticking to a low-fat diet to guard against heart attack and obesity can then put you at risk of osteoporosis, which cheese, butter and milk would help to avoid. Skimmed and low-fat milk *are* as high in calcium as full-fat, and it may be worth edging towards one evil to avoid another. Calcium is also found in fortified soya milk (available from healthfood shops), in fish with the bones intact, such as whitebait or tinned pilchards and sardines, and in 'hard' water. So if you live in a hard-water area it may not be an advantage to fit a water softener to your supply or to filter your drinking water through such a device. Whether you opt for being slim or cuddly can also provide you with a dilemma at menopause. It is the stopping of oestrogen-production by the ovaries that causes all the trouble. After menopause, the adrenal glands continue to manufacture a form of this hormone that can be converted into oestrogen while being stored in fat deposits in the body. The greater your fat stores, the more oestrogen you convert. This is why fat and jolly old ladies often have such youthful, smooth skin. However, they are also at risk of all the hazards of being overweight, so it is a case of paying your money and taking your choice!

Alternatively, discuss with your doctor the possibility of trying hormone replacement therapy (HRT) for a time. In HRT, artificial hormones are used and have the effect of both keeping menopausal symptoms at bay and preventing calcium shedding. Indeed, the effect is protective for some time after therapy has stopped, so a few years on HRT significantly delay calcium loss. HRT also protects against ischaemic heart disease that lessens the blood-supply to the heart. HRT is usually recommended to continue for two years if the reasons for needing it were symptoms such as hot flushes, while it can continue for longer if the cause was vaginal dryness. Originally, HRT consisted of giving unopposed oestrogen, which led to an increased risk to women with intact wombs of developing cancer of the endometrium. Now, HRT includes progestogen and this successfully prevents such a risk. However, some women and some doctors still feel uneasy about HRT, perhaps on the grounds that it is 'unnatural' or only asked for by vain women. In the United States, it was originally heralded as the pill promising eternal youth! Only 2 per cent of women in the UK are prescribed HRT, while the figure in the States is 30 per cent. It has been suggested that this has a lot to do with the fact that American women are 'customers' rather than 'patients' and can demand a treatment they feel is worthwhile. Some women do find the fact that being on HRT means you continue to have periods somewhat off-putting. The various pros and cons of treatment are something you and your doctor would have to discuss.

## TALKING TO YOUR DOCTOR

If you are going to take responsibility for your health while you are well, and do your best to ensure that you stay that way, you may also find it logical to ask for more of a say when you are ill. Your doctor might have the expertise to know what is wrong and what should be done, but ultimately, since it is your body, you should have the final word. You cannot do this unless you know what is happening to your body. When we see a doctor, therefore, we must get into the habit of asking as much as possible about the situation. If you find that you tend to 'go blank' when you see your doctor, and emerge with a prescription but very little understanding of what it is for, or have been sent away with reassurance that does *not* reassure because you cannot remember a single thing that was said, try these strategies. List your questions before you go, so you will not forget any of them. Make sure you go through the whole list, and if your doctor seems at all unwilling to explain fully, say, 'You are obviously busy now, so I will make an appointment to come back at a better time, to allow you to give me a proper explanation.' The key questions anyone needs answered when seeing a doctor are:

Is something wrong?
What is wrong and with what part of my body?
How serious is it?
What will happen?
What treatment is needed, either from you or from me?
If you give me tablets, how and when should I take them?
How will they work, what side-effects could they have?
How can I make sure this condition will not return?

Doctors are not there to tell you what to do – how to live, how to love and how to behave. They have no real training to allow them to be moral mentors and no right to corner the market on *any* aspect of information. They do, however, have years of experience in recognizing, diagnosing and treating illness. The key to a successful and healthy life is recognizing that your health is ultimately your own responsibility, but knowing which aspects should be left to you and which should be taken to your doctor. Once there, you need to be firm as to which is your field and which is his or hers. The ideal is a partnership, and most doctors now welcome having patients who come with a certain amount of self-awareness and knowledge, and who want to communicate and learn.

# CHAPTER 5

# The Men
# In Your Life

There is no doubt that many people find the idea of women doing self-examination alarming. The reasons usually given, however, do not stand up to examination. Would we hurt ourselves? No more than we might with tampons or toothpicks, yet we are trusted with those. And if this were a good reason, then surely the obvious answer would be to encourage us to learn how to do it properly so that we would not be at risk? Would we be able to make any sense of what we found? Such an argument seems to suggest that you need seven years of medical training to be able to notice when a discharge that is usually cream-coloured is now green or bloodstained – not exactly a defensible idea. Self-examination does not imply self-diagnosis and treatment, but is suggested as a way of monitoring our own health so that we know when to ask for the skilled services of the professionals.

When we cut through the rhetoric against women taking possession of their own bodies, we come up against the deep emotional reaction experienced by many men towards such activity. If you intend to follow the suggestions in this book, you may need to understand and take account of these, for you might find opposition, ridicule or anxiety displayed by the men with whom you come into contact, whether sexual partners, fathers or doctors. And you may also find their attitudes mirrored in some areas of the Establishment.

The largest high street chemist refuses to sell speculums to women unless they can offer a letter from their doctor 'permitting' the purchase. In contrast, the British Medical Association enthusiastically supports women learning about their bodies in any way they can. As the representative of all GPs, they say that very few of their members would disagree with this, and that the official guidelines are not in favour of putting barriers in women's way. In spite of this, the chemist's medical advisers insist on the ban.

## BARRIERS

Why *do* men find women's self-examination challenging? Perhaps it is because self-examination does appear somewhat extraordinary. Very few of us are supple enough to view our genitals without the aid of a mirror and torch. Even if we could look unaided, it still needs a contortionist's skills. Such a carry-on makes the act seem unusual and even abnormal. Men can, and do, touch and look at *their* genitals every day. But since it requires no unusual effort, this passes unnoticed and unremarked. The effort we have to invest makes the act seem wrong as well as ludicrous.

Men touch themselves regularly, to pass water – a routine act that 'normalizes' their handling of themselves. Women touch themselves for only two reasons – during menstruation and masturbation. Both these are surrounded by taboo and myth and this colours any other handling.

Menstruation has been a frightening phenomenon for centuries. Only women can bleed without there being an obvious wound and women's menstrual blood is a source of fear and ritual in many societies. Women are also supposed to be 'innocent'. Masturbation is often a source of guilt for men, but it is even more frowned on in girls, since girls are expected to be passive when it comes to sexual knowledge and sexual activity. One of the greatest slurs on a young girl's character is the accusation that she is 'too knowing' when it comes to sex, or that 'she wants it'. Since most genital touching takes place in sexual contact and is done *by* men, it is hard for men to divorce the act from its sexual overtones. It is hard for men not to see such touching as trespassing on *their* territory. Sexual pleasure is seen as a gift men bestow on women, and for women to explore their own bodies is for them to seek to reject this gift by taking it over.

The vagina holds as many mysteries for men as it does for women, if not more. It is largely unseen and the extreme sensitivity of our fingers multiplies the apparently roughened, irregular nature of this area. Female genitals, unlike male, are moist. Although as small children we all revelled in the sensuous pleasures of squidgy mud or running water, we were usually told off for 'getting dirty'. So, what is instinctively an intensely pleasant sensation could have unpleasant associations for many of us.

There is another barrier. The words we use to describe sexual contact are often surprisingly violent. Men 'have' or possess women. In sexual excitement they are said to be 'horny', and their penis is a 'prick' or 'prong'. The fears that men have of their womenfolk doing damage to themselves, or *finding* damage, are therefore understandable. Men often harbour fears about their partner's genitals. They may think that this area is extremely vulnerable and liable to be damaged by them – men whose partners develop infections or diseases in the reproductive organs often blame themselves, but are unable to express their feelings. Or they may become convinced that the vagina holds risks for them, and can crush or hurt them.

A man's own ignorance may also be a barrier. If he himself is puzzled and in the dark about a subject, he may be resentful of the idea of someone else knowing more than he does, especially when he feels that the subject is one over which he has more right to be informed. If he sees his sexual partner's genitals as *his* territory, this may be how he feels. We are often encouraged to see sexuality as a mystery, and all the more exciting for that. Seeking knowledge can be seen as threatening that mystery and therefore being undesirable. Conversely, many men see information about 'women's matters' as being nothing to do with them. The fact that family planning clinics and Well Woman centres are female-only territory serves to strengthen this ghetto-izing. When barred from an area, whether physical or conceptual, it is human nature to respond with an aggressive, 'Well, I didn't really want to go there anyway!'

The medical profession adds a further layer to this opposition. Not only are the majority of doctors male, with all the uncertainties and fears of their sex, they are also professionals with a job to protect. They see the sexual areas of a woman's body as their preserve, and regard knowledge about them as the exclusive property of their profession.

You may well find that your own partner is delighted that you are going to take care of yourself by monitoring your own health. If you see your own doctor, you may discover yours is one who is happy to have you take such responsibility. If neither is the case, what should you do?

## AVOIDANCE

One strategy is simple avoidance. You can bring up the subject, but if it meets with hostility, drop it and go your own way without discussing it again. Find times when you are assured of privacy to do your monitoring, and keep any equipment necessary out of sight. If you do see your doctor as the result of a symptom spotted during a check, say instead that you just happened to notice it.

There are enormous drawbacks to such an approach. For a start, it is extremely difficult to keep secrets from a close companion. It can make them suspicious, and you resentful. Since you never impress them with the importance of what you are doing, and never relieve the mystery, it will always be a source of fear and conflict. A lack of honesty on your part means he has no reason to come clean on his. He may not share information with you about his own past and present health that could have a significant bearing on your health care.

Not telling a doctor about your actions would leave a good doctor missing vital clues. If you arrive with a symptom but don't explain how and why you noticed it, and that your regular monitoring gives you good reason to be alarmed, the doctor may not take as much notice as he or she should. A bad doctor, who is resentful of self-examination, will be left unchallenged, never seeing the value of what you do.

## DISCUSSION

Another strategy, then, is to discuss the matter with the men in your life, but continue to do your own monitoring in private. By explanation and demonstration of the results, you can try to convince them that what you are doing makes excellent sense and is normal. This approach has many benefits. However convinced you are of the necessity of doing health checks, you may still prefer to carry them out on your own. Most of us feel fairly vulnerable when naked, and it is easy to feel a little foolish when crouching over a mirror, or to think that it looks a bit vain to be peering at your breasts. If, however, you are clear that you intend to do this, you can bring any fears or hostilities out into the open. Quite a few men will be pleased and relieved you *are* looking after yourself, but may not want to be involved themselves. They may have a lingering feeling that genitals are basically ugly and not want to look closely at them. Or they may be afraid that if they look dispassionately, they will lose the ability to become aroused at sexual moments. They may be afraid of making a fool of themselves by becoming aroused at an inappropriate time! However, if you explain why it is important, they may be willing to talk about any sexual behaviour of their own that could put you at risk. They may also be willing to take their own steps to help both of you achieve good health, separately and together. This might be in joining in physical exercise and eating a balanced diet. It could be in examining unhealthy practices such as drinking too much or smoking. It could be in discussing with an employer, union representative or a doctor whether their workplace or working conditions puts them at risk. It could also be in applying some of your lessons to themselves.

## SELF-EXAMINATION FOR MEN

Self-examination is just as important for men as it is for women. Strange as it may seem, men suffer from breast cancer as well. Only 1 to 2 per cent of deaths from this disease occur in men – but men who do develop malignant tumours are far more likely to die from this disease than women. The reason is that even fewer men than women detect a lump in this area and seek help. Just as with women, men should get into the regular habit of running the flats of their fingers around the fleshy area surrounding the nipple, and into the armpit. Once a month, after a shower or bath, is a good interval, and 'his and hers' simultaneous health checks could be an excellent memory jogger for both of you.

At the same time, men should take the opportunity to search for any suspicious lumps in the testicles. Testicular cancer is rare in that it accounts for only 1 to 2 per cent of all cancers in men. However, it is the most common cancer to strike *young* men. Like cancer of the cervix in women, if detected early enough it is relatively easy to treat and can be cured without long-lasting damage.

Testicular checks are best done standing up, after a warm bath, when the scrotum is relaxed. Starting on one side, index and middle fingers are placed under one testicle, the thumb on top, and the testicle rolled gently between them. It should feel firm – a bit like an earlobe – but have some 'give'. There should not be any hard lumps or swellings. If one is found, whether it is painful or not, this should be shown to a doctor as soon as possible. Testicular tumours are

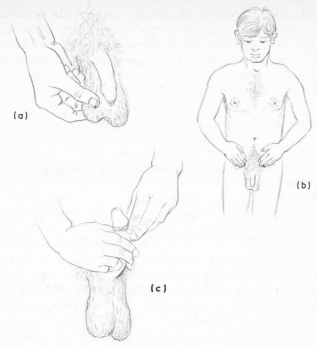

Male self-examination: *a* feeling the testicles; *b* feeling in the groin; *c* examining
the glans

usually malignant and liable to spread and form secondary tumours,
so they do need to be treated quickly. Sometimes the scrotum appears
to enlarge, rather than there being a clear lump. A man who has
become used to examining himself will notice any changes in shape,
size, sensitivity or consistency. With the flats of the fingers, the area
above and to each side of the genitals, in the groin, should be felt for
any lumps or tender spots. While resting hands on the area, he
should cough to see if any bump becomes apparent. Testicular cancer
can show itself in other ways before a lump or swelling becomes
noticeable, so a dull ache in the lower abdomen, pain in the lower
back or a dragging, heavy feeling in this area should always be
reported to a doctor. To finish, the penis should also be examined for
any signs of discharge or sores. Pulling back the foreskin, the end of
the penis and opening to the urethra should be looked at. Men whose
partners have abnormal smears should be screened by their doctors.

Cancer cannot be caught or passed on from one person to the other, but it may be found that one of the causative elements in a woman developing cancerous changes was wart virus. If the man has this, treatment will be necessary to protect both partners. Wart virus may increase the risks of developing penile cancer as well as cervical cancer.

## INVOLVEMENT

Some men might welcome the opportunity to become more involved in your explorations. Self-examination *is* easier if you have an extra pair of hands to hold the mirror or light source and to tilt them if necessary. While you are learning to appreciate and know your own body, so can he. A chance to see inside the vagina, using a speculum, and to gently feel the walls other than during intercourse, can dispel any fears he might have about the vulnerability of your sexual parts or sexuality in the face of his male 'rapaciousness', or the risks his tender organ might run inside you. Not only can this increase his understanding of your body, it can lead to an increase in your pleasure in each other. By looking at each other's genitals, you can soon appreciate that this part of the body is not ugly or unpleasant, just unfamiliar. Familiarity, instead of breeding contempt, engenders understanding and appreciation.

Most women might like to see it as their responsibility to pass on the habit of getting to know and looking after ourselves to any daughter they might have, and to friends and relatives who could benefit from learning the value of such activity. If you were able to help the man in your life to accept and see the value of self-examination, this would become the attitude *they* would pass on to the next male generation. Nothing succeeds like success, so the more you demonstrate the undeniable benefits of looking after yourself and understanding yourself, the more easily the men in your life can accept and learn the point of it all.

# CHAPTER 6

# *Contraception*

W ell Woman care often begins with, and subsequently focuses around, a visit to a doctor or clinic for birth-control. The exercise of our sexuality and the health of our sexual and reproductive parts become linked. This can cause problems. It is easy to imagine that any ill health in these areas must be a result of our sexual activities and practices. Sexual love, which should be a normal and joyful part of our lives and relationships, can become fraught with guilt and fear. Even if we are happy in our behaviour, we fear – rightly, in many cases – censure and disdain from the professionals who are supposed to help us. This fear can be a barrier to our asking for their help.

The link is difficult to break because it is often very logical. Although Well Woman care is something you can do for yourself from a very early age, and many of the measures you or your medical carers should take to maintain your health have nothing to do with this part of your life, a first visit to a doctor for birth-control is often the best time for you to be brought into the system of cervical and breast checks. Before then, you may not be old enough for monitoring to show anything of value and, of course, the very start of sexual relationships that makes contraception necessary also puts us at certain risks.

Contraception, however, has further implications than just being the 'calling card' to get us into Well Woman care. If you see such care as giving you control and an appreciation of yourself and your life, the choice and use of a method of birth-control can be a central part of this empowerment.

Just as people often choose a new outfit, a new car, job or even life-partner without real consideration, simply by picking what is on display that day, many of us get burdened with an unsuitable method of birth-control because we allow very little *real* choice to be made. If you want your contraception to be right, you need to ask yourself certain questions. The most important of these is – what do I want from a method of birth-control?

The answer appears obvious. As the name implies, the purpose of contraception is to prevent pregnancy. Reflecting this, any literature on the subject – whether newspaper or magazine articles, explanatory leaflets or books – tends to take efficiency as the most important aspect of each method. When doctors, nurses, and agony aunties are asked, 'What is the *best* method?' they know that what is meant is, 'Which has the lowest pregnancy rate?' Drug companies sponsoring research into new methods all emphasize what has been called 'the crazy pursuit of the nought per cent pregnancy rate'.

Crazy? Yes, because in spite of a stated preoccupation with efficiency, actual contraceptive behaviour shows, and has been showing for some years, that for both men and women, prevention of pregnancy may *not* be the most important aspect of a contraceptive method.

The failure rates of contraceptives have always been a matter of debate. Drug companies and researchers are quick to explain that variations between trials arise from 'user' rather than 'method' failure. The implication is that a difference in pregnancy rate between a trial composed of middle-class white Americans and working-class Puerto Ricans is due to lack of education, understanding and motivation on the part of one of the groups.

Fleming nearly threw away a nasty mould which formed on a failed experiment before realizing he had inadvertently discovered something useful (he called it penicillin). Similarly, evidence from several apparently abortive studies is not so much being deliberately suppressed as innocently disregarded. Yet this could, and should, shed light on what users *really* value in birth-control.

The Margaret Pyke Clinic in London started a trial in 1980 on the contraceptive sponge. Eventually 250 women were recruited, of which half used the sponge and half acted as controls using a conventional diaphragm and spermicide. Large-scale American trials had produced pregnancy rates similar to those found with a diaphragm. As the UK trial drew to a close at the end of 1983, the pregnancy rate for sponge users was twice that of diaphragm users, in spite of the subjects being professional women with high motivation. But when told that the trial was ending and no more supplies of the sponge would be available, women begged to be allowed to continue with the method – even when told of the high pregnancy rate.

At the same time, doctors at Marie Stopes House were carrying out a similar but less formal study on diaphragm use. Following the theory of an American gynaecologist, women coming into the clinic for a diaphragm were offered the NSFFC (non-spermicidal fit free cap). This is a small version which is worn continuously, only being removed once a day for cleaning. One size fits everyone, and it is used without spermicide. The study was discontinued by the supervising doctor because of her dismay at the high pregnancy rate. Again, women positively begged to be allowed to continue with the method, even when given the reasons for the discontinuation of the trial.

The connection between these two methods is their marked lack of fuss and 'mess'. In using the NSFFC, you do away with all the bother of having to anticipate sex, especially the necessity to make sure that spermicides are used and inserted no more than two hours before making love. With the sponge, not only can you forget spermicides, but it even soaks up semen itself. No more arguing about who sleeps on the damp patch!

Voice such a concern to your family planning doctor, and you may find yourself marked down as having a psychosexual problem. A dislike of the diaphragm can be interpreted as being the result of a Victorian upbringing or an unhealthy obsession with hygiene. And any distaste or dissatisfaction with the paraphernalia of contraception is usually taken as a symptom of a neurotic personality or a crumbling relationship.

Undoubtedly, this *can* be true. Some of us see ourselves as mothers, not individuals, with the ability to procreate as our only or main asset. Contraception thus threatens our role in life. Some of us, ambivalent towards our sexuality, can only allow sex to happen *to* us, rather than by a conscious decision. Using contraception, particularly a method such as a cap, which requires affirmation of our sexuality before every sexual act, or the Pill, which requires acknowledgement of sexual intention each day, means having to declare ourselves as sexual beings. For teenagers, especially, this may be difficult. Others use dissatisfaction with a method, or a refusal to use one, as a means of signalling the end of a relationship. The rejection of the Pill as no longer being 'safe' or giving you a headache may be a statement about your sexual partner.

Some men and women use birth-control – or the lack of it – to gain and keep control over their partner's or even their own sexual desires. Thus, the insecure man may insist on his using the sheath or withdrawal in the belief that his wife cannot safely take a lover. Or, indeed, so that he can have the accident-on-purpose and keep her 'barefoot and pregnant'. By not using a method, the insecure woman who finds no pleasure in sex can always reject advances on the grounds that, 'It's not my safe time'. In many cases, it cannot be denied that difficulties with birth-control are symptomatic of deeper problems. But it could be argued that a neurotic reaction is one which is out of step. When a particular reaction is virtually a universal response, it is time to consider whether the label of 'neurotic' is wrong, rather than the behaviour itself.

It is a pity that an Edward De Bono has not applied some lateral thinking to the problem of birth-control acceptability. As yet, everyone concentrates on the same line:

1. Birth-control is there to prevent births. Therefore:
2. When it fails it's because users are being irrational/lazy/stupid. Therefore:
3. Try to make it more efficient and foolproof.

Hardly any studies have moved off sideways to explore:

1. *Why* people find methods unacceptable.
2. *What* we find unacceptable and *why* these factors should be more important than the fear of pregnancy.

Above all, in our society we put contraception in the mental context of long-term planning: 'If I use a sheath/cap/pill now, I'll be glad in nine months' time when I won't have another mouth to feed.' But where does delayed gratification come in the sexual act? You make love because you want to feel pleasure, show love or share sensation *now*. Unless sex is happening because a child is wanted (and deliberate sex-for-pregnancy is far rarer than pregnancy-as-a-side-effect-of-sex), the consequences of the act are irrelevant at the time. Uppermost in lovers' minds are the immediate emotional or physical benefits. Sex makes you feel good, lets you show affection and allows you to feel masculine or feminine. Which is why the immediate and certain emotional or physical drawbacks of a birth-control method become so much more important, *at the time*, than the future possible drawbacks of unwanted pregnancy. If the method is unpleasant or detracts from your fun, or makes you fear for your health, one of two things is likely to happen. Either you will not use it or you will find that your concern or distaste spoils all enjoyment.

Cultural attitudes towards birth-control methods are known and allowed for when they appear in 'primitive' or non-Western societies. Depo-Provera, for instance, is known as a widely tolerated method in areas such as North Thailand in spite of any side-effects, because, after government health drives, injections are associated with better health. The Pill, on the other hand, is virtually unused in Japan because pill-taking is seen as 'illness' behaviour. An IUCD that was widely accepted in the Western world – the Lippes Loop – was a total failure in India because it tends to increase menstrual bleeding. This bleeding was inside the range of acceptability of the biomedical scientists offering the method, but intolerable to Indian women. But it seems easier for doctors to label similar 'irrational' behaviour in members of a First World country as neurotic, rather than to accept it as a universal human reaction – and allow for it.

In one of the few studies to investigate attitudes to contraceptive methods, Canberra University Psychological Department, used a semantic test on 172 sexually active students, both male and female. The test was designed to gauge their gut reaction to forty pairs of adjectives describing ten methods – Pill, IUCD, condom, diaphragm, male and female sterilization, spermicides, douches, rhythm and withdrawal. The paired adjectives included 'non-messy – messy', 'attractive – ugly', 'non-embarrassing – embarrassing', 'pleasurable – unpleasant', 'non-distressful – distressful' and 'quick – time-consuming'. The words presented covered concepts one might consider important when thinking of contraception.

There were seven basic attributes: effectiveness and reliability; discretion and modesty; pleasure, mood or aesthetics; legality and morality; permanence and flexibility; health and harmfulness; time or cost. Men and women largely agreed on scores, although for women, excitement and pleasure were more important than discretion and unobtrusiveness. Mood was very significant to women as was comfort, although men were little concerned about this. Both were more concerned about 'mess' than about health risks. Spermicides received one of the highest negative scores for being a 'messy' method, as well as being 'distressful', 'uncomfortable' and 'ugly'. The sheath, too, scored high on ugliness and distressfulness, as well as being labelled 'unnatural' and 'visible'.

Your sexual partner's attitude towards your method of contraception is as important as your own. You may sabotage your own successful use of a method by being ambivalent towards its use. Your partner's hostility to a method you find acceptable can be just as devastating. Women can find their lover's use of a condom insulting or laughable; men can find the use of a diaphragm unaesthetic or excluding. The other person's use of birth-control can also be seen as a threat to your femininity or masculinity and potency. A high failure rate has been found to go hand in hand with the objection by a partner to a particular method or general use.

Before a method of contraception can be acquired and used, a complex process of decision-making has to be undergone. For a start, the potential user has to admit to themselves that they *are* having sex and risk causing or suffering pregnancy. The inhibited, the embarrassed or the young may prefer to believe that sex is not something they are choosing to do – it happens without their prior knowledge and consent and they 'can't help it'. The comforting myth that pregnancy happens only to 'bad' girls is part of the denial of sexual feelings. At the same time, the potential user must be able to accept that he or she *can* take control of their own life. To many women, not only sex but life happens *to* them and they view their existence and any possibilities of pregnancy with a certain fatalism.

Even if it is accepted that the risk is real and could be avoided, the pros and cons of using or not using contraception have to be weighed up. The drawbacks of unplanned or unwanted pregnancy may seem obvious – an extra mouth to feed, loss of earnings or education, curtailment of social life, stigma and parental disappointment if the girl is young or unmarried. But against that can be set the *advantages*. Motherhood conveys status, attention and an object to love and be loved by. A pregnancy will prove the maturity and the masculinity or femininity of the parents and test a relationship. Most important perhaps are the 'costs' of using a method of birth-control. Contraception may prevent pregnancy, but all methods are embarrassing and troublesome to obtain, unpleasant or inconvenient to use and most get in the way of what the majority of people consider to be the real business of sex, which is spontaneous pleasure with no after-effects. To many, the 'cost' of contraception is too high.

Many of life's pleasures are heightened by anticipation. The spontaneous picnic, midnight swim or meal out may have their place, but what can be more delightful than an eagerly awaited and meticulously planned treat? Except, of course, when it comes to sex, where the majority of us still vote with our genitals in insisting that preparation and expectation are immoral or cold-blooded.

A further question that has to be asked when making your choice of method is, 'Am I trying to come to a decision from a full range of methods, and is it *my* convenience that is being considered or my doctor's?' Some methods are not available from your family doctor. Condoms, for instance, can only be prescribed on the NHS by clinics, or bought in shops. Many doctors do not have the necessary training or the practice necessary for them to fit an IUCD. Some family doctors will prefer to prescribe the Pill rather than other methods, because doing so is quicker and easier than fiddling about with the explanations and fittings of other methods. The doctors may not even realize this is what they are doing, but explain their bias in terms of its being the 'best' choice for you. What may get lost is how you *feel* about this choice, which is not one made freely, and how it affects your later actions.

Having explored what we want from a method of contraception and made ourselves aware of how our partners and medical advisers may feel, the next stage is to become familiar with all the methods. To make a free choice, you need to know what is available and how to use it.

## CONTRACEPTIVE METHODS THAT HINDER ——— SEXUAL ACTIVITY ———

There are two methods of contraception that work by affecting when or how you make love.

### PERIODIC ABSTINENCE

This is also known as the rhythm method, the safe period, or 'Vatican roulette'. The user abstains from sex at the times in her menstrual cycle when she is most likely to conceive. At its simplest level, this is used by the teenager who avoids sex in a haphazard manner somewhere midway between her periods, when ovulation is most likely to occur. At its most complex level, couples can use a variety of techniques to pinpoint ovulation fairly accurately and abstain for several days before and after this event.

There are four basic ways of finding out when ovulation is likely to occur – the temperature method, the mucus or Billings method, the calendar method and ovulation testing.

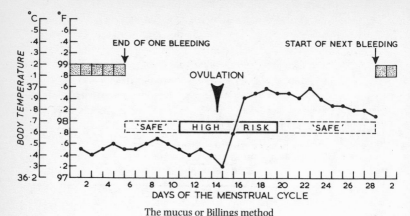

The mucus or Billings method

### The temperature method

Just before ovulation, your temperature is likely to drop very slightly and then rise until a few days before your next period. You can see this progression if you take and note down your temperature each morning *before* getting up or doing anything to raise it (such as having a hot drink or making love). After three consecutive days at the raised temperature, you will be safe to have sex since ovulation will have occurred and by this time the egg will have decayed to a point where it is unlikely to be fertilized. If you keep a regular chart and your cycle is extremely stable, you may well feel confident enough to work out which days in the cycle are safe *before* ovulation is likely to happen. Since sperm can survive for as much as five days and even in the most regular cycle ovulation can happen earlier than you expect, you may only be able to allow yourself between one and four days after your period has stopped. Strictly speaking, the only 'safe' time in the temperature method is *after* ovulation. In a regular twenty-eight-day cycle, this would amount to around ten days each month.

If you want to pursue this method, you would be advised to discuss it with your own doctor or one at a family planning clinic, and to use the special free thermometer and charts they can give you. Note also that your temperature can be raised by illness and lowered by medicines such as aspirin – so be on the lookout for inaccurate readings.

### The mucus or Billing method

Unlike the temperature method, successful use of the mucus method

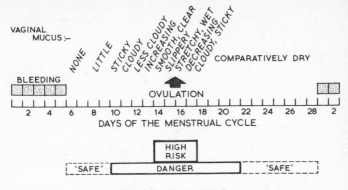

The temperature method

gives you some early warning signals of the approach of ovulation. Three to four days before an egg is released, your body begins to ready itself for impregnation. The cervix releases a flow of mucus which mingles with the regular flow of liquid from the walls of the vagina. Vaginal secretions are opaque and somewhat thick. This new wetness is clear, stretchy and thin. The cervical mucus is designed to help sperm on its way through the cervical canal and on up the womb into the fallopian tubes.

Users of this method should avoid intercourse from as soon as they notice an increase in vaginal wetness until they have been relatively dry again for four days. A further test for whether the increase *is* due to cervical mucus, rather than just an increase in the amount of vaginal fluid being produced, is to rub a small amount between two fingers and then separate them. If the fluid is slippery and elastic in texture, and stretches for a few centimetres before breaking, it is likely to be pre-ovulatory cervical mucus. However, if your cycle is short, you may find that the warning change happens during or just after your period and so can be missed.

### The calendar method

In the calendar method, you chart your periods over a time and use that information to predict the probable 'safe' days. However, even women who think they have a regular cycle are likely to find that each month is slightly different. Periods are likely to come on from between twenty-five to thirty-two days after the previous bleed. This

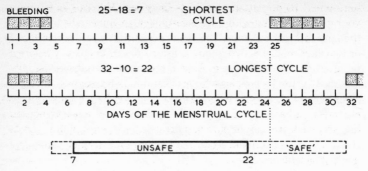

The calendar method

makes anticipating the next ovulation a bit difficult. The day on which you release an egg is not affected by when you had your *last* bleed – it can come four or fourteen days afterwards. It is, however, linked to when you have your *next* period, since it is ovulation itself that sets in train the changes that lead up to this event. Ovulation is almost always followed by a period fourteen days later. However, even this *can* be delayed or speeded up by two days.

In the calendar method, you keep a record of the first day of your period for at least six – preferably twelve – months. The aim then is to predict the likely spread of the safe and unsafe days in subsequent months. You do this by taking the *shortest* cycle, say twenty-five days, and subtract from it the figure eighteen. In this case, that gives you seven. You then take the longest cycle, say thirty-two days, and take from it the figure ten. In this case, you are left with twenty-two. This would mean that your first unsafe day in any cycle is likely to be seven days after the beginning of your period, and your last unsafe day is likely to be twenty-two days after the beginning of your last period. To be safe from pregnancy, you can only make love up until the sixth day after a period starts, and on the twenty-third day onwards. Of course, in a twenty-five-day cycle in which your bleeding lasts for seven days, this would allow you only two days of sex if you or your partner dislikes having intercourse during menstruation.

## Ovulation testing

You can buy special kits from a chemist that claim to predict when ovulation is due. These work on the fact that one or two days before ovulation takes place, the amount of a hormone called luteinising hormone (LH) present in your body increases. This can be found in your urine by testing with a special sampler, so you can be warned of the approach of ovulation. The drawback is that you have only one or two days' notice of ovulation, so intercourse immediately before a positive test is very likely to make you pregnant. The kits are actually intended for use by couples who are planning a pregnancy, and give an excellent indication of when to make love to enhance your chances of starting a baby. Since they enable you to know when ovulation has occurred, you can be sure you are safe for the rest of the month. However, in their present form, the kits are an extremely expensive method of contraception.

## Combinations of methods

The most effective option is to combine several of these methods, taking your temperature but also watching for changes in mucus and other signs such as Mittelschmerz to indicate ovulation is about to happen or has happened. Used with care and will-power, safe-period methods can be as much as 85 to 93 per cent effective – that is, used by 100 women over a year, between seven and fifteen women will become pregnant using them. However, they can also be little better than useless – hence the name Vatican roulette, and the remark by one family planning expert: 'There is a name for people who use the rhythm method – parents.' The calendar method used on its own is suggested to have an efficiency rating of only 53 per cent.

As the term 'periodic abstinence' suggests, the point of all these elaborate charts and observations is to find out when would be the most likely time of the month for you to conceive, and to avoid having sex on these days. Enthusiastic users of the method claim several advantages for it. There are no physical side-effects or health risks and the method is accepted by religions and cultures that otherwise frown on birth-control. The method is under the couple's personal control, and once established is always available – even when chemists and doctors' surgeries are closed. The communication and closeness necessary to make such a method work are said to bring a couple together, and restricting sex to certain days gives it the spice of anticipation.

Periodic abstinence can be particularly successful for the mature, confident and stable couple who can make what would be a detraction for a young person a plus in their relationship. The over thirty-fives can benefit from the fact that their fertility is less than it was ten or twenty years before. Calculating the safe period becomes difficult as menopause approaches and periods become irregular, however, so this method may not be practical for the older couple. Temperature charts, special thermometers and training on using all these methods are available from your own family doctor or practice nurse, a nurse or doctor at a family planning clinic or from the Catholic Marriage Advisory Council.

## COITUS INTERRUPTUS

The second method that affects love-making is coitus interruptus, also known as withdrawal, 'pulling out' or 'being careful'. In this, the man withdraws his penis before ejaculation and 'comes' or has his orgasm outside his partner. The idea is that, by not depositing semen inside her, there is no risk of pregnancy. It is probably the oldest method of birth-control, apart from infanticide and abortion.

Coitus interruptus has a bad reputation and the main disadvantage is said to be its inefficiency. Living sperm can be found in the lubricating fluid that oozes from the penis *before* ejaculation. By the time the man withdraws, sperm may already be on its way towards a meeting with the ovum. However, various studies of the method do not appear to bear this out. Among highly motivated couples, the failure rate from withdrawal can be the same as the failure rate from mechanical means of contraception, such as diaphragms. As with most methods, the key seems to be whether or not the users are happy to employ it and are confident and practised.

The advantages of withdrawal are that it requires no external preparation at all – no chart, no pills, no bits and pieces. It cannot be lost, forgotten when you go away or left off the shopping list. It has no physical side-effects. Its critics claim that – as with periodic abstinence – the method causes stress. Pulling out makes the experience incomplete for the man and unsatisfactory for the woman. Furthermore, fear of pregnancy means that the woman is unable to relax and enjoy love-making at all. Most of all, the critics complain, the worst drawback is that the method doesn't work.

All of this may be true when the method is used hastily by an inexperienced couple, and not as the result of a decision but because they have no other method to hand. Its failures, then, are a result of a general lack of experience and communication. *If* the couple agrees that this is to be their chosen method, practise its use so that the man *does* pull out in time and makes sure that the female partner is sexually satisfied, there is no reason why the method need be totally unsatisfactory. Methods which affect love-making itself, either by making it untenable at certain times or interrupted each time, are acceptable to some people and this fact should be accepted by all of us.

Fear of AIDS has meant that many people have changed their attitudes to what is 'normal' or 'desirable' sexual practice. Up to now, the understanding has been that sexual expression consists of a man and a woman caressing each other as a prelude to 'the real thing', and that this is the insertion of the penis into the vagina. Once in, thrusting movements result in a satisfying and preferably simultaneous climax for both partners, which ends the encounter. In practice, most couples have always made variations on this theme – involving oral sex, mutual masturbation and, in some cases, anal penetration. The majority of women do not have an orgasm from straight, man-on-top penetrative sex but find that clitoral stimulation from hands, lips or tongue or from the woman-on-top position is needed for full mutual enjoyment. The necessary medical advice that exchange of body fluids should be avoided has led many couples to find that penetrative sex is not the 'be-all-and-end-all' of sex. By giving each other pleasure by using every other part of their bodies except genital-to-genital exchanges, many couples have found that avoiding the depositing of semen inside the woman need not be a chore, but can be a natural part of even more exciting sex than intercourse. For this reason, withdrawal as a method of birth control may soon be seen in a more positive light.

## CONTRACEPTIVE METHODS USED AT THE TIME OF ——— MAKING LOVE ———

There are five methods that can be used just before, during or after love-making. These are the four 'barrier' methods of condom, cap or diaphragm, sponge and spermicide, and douching.

### THE CONDOM

The condom or sheath is a thin rubber tube, designed to cover the penis during love-making and to contain the man's semen after

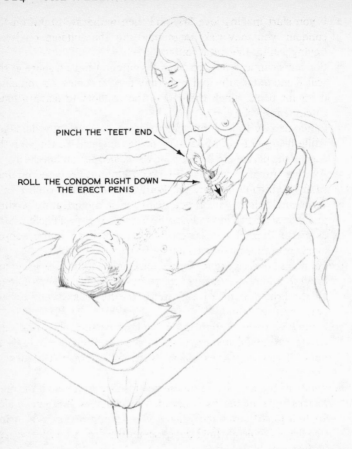

PINCH THE 'TEET' END

ROLL THE CONDOM RIGHT DOWN
THE ERECT PENIS

Putting on a condom

climax. The condom can be put on by the man or his partner, or they can do it together. Condoms come packed in threes or dozens, and each individual condom is sealed in its own foil or plastic wrapper. The thin tube is closed off at one end, the open end having a firm rim or ring – like that on the mouth of a balloon. Condoms come rolled up, and the idea is that you place one on the end of the erect penis and unroll the device down its length like putting on a rolled-up stocking. Important points to note in condom use are:

1. A condom can really only be put on an excited and erect penis.

2. If you start making love first and then withdraw to put on the condom, you may risk pregnancy. Put the condom on *before* having genital-to-genital contact.

3. Condoms can leak or even burst if you don't have a space at the sealed end to take the man's sperm when he comes. As you place it on his penis, pinch the end of the condom to leave a loose catchment space.

4. Condoms can leak or burst if they are even slightly damaged while being put on. Make sure ragged fingernails, rings or the edge of the packaging do not snag the device as you handle it.

5. Another threat to the sheath is the use of any oil-based product such as vaseline or baby oil. Both can perish the rubber in a surprisingly short time. If you want to use a lubricating product to aid or add extra fun to love-making, use the special jellies such as KY or Durex Lubricating jelly for vaginal use, and a non-oil massage or moisturizing cream for the rest of your body.

6. Condoms are designed to be used once only – it is a false economy to wash and re-use them – and you are strongly advised to look for the British Standard 'Kite mark' on the package and to buy only approved brands.

7. Using two condoms at once does *not* improve their efficiency – the two layers rub against each other and both condoms are likely to burst. If you want extra safety, there are 'stronger' varieties on sale.

8. Condoms can slip off and spill semen inside the woman if the man relaxes and remains inside her after he climaxes. It is a good idea for him to withdraw fairly soon after having his orgasm, using two fingers to firmly hold the condom in place as he does so – or for her to do it for him.

Condoms do suffer from an image problem. They have been used for centuries as a protection from STDs and many of us still associate them with disease and illicit sex. Men and women can be put off buying supplies for fear of the reactions of the person behind the counter or their sexual partner. Men can be particularly frightened of using one in case their awkward fumbling suggests inexperience. Men are *supposed* to be experts when it comes to sex, while women are reluctant to show knowledge in case the offer of a condom suggests too much experience – women are *supposed* to be innocent in sexual matters. Men might also refuse to use a condom on the grounds that it spoils their pleasure – a claim very much out of date with new materials that can be made into an extraordinarily thin product. In reality, their dread is often that they might lose an erection while trying to put on the device, or trigger a premature ejaculation by handling themselves. It's a sad fact that very few boys or men will plan ahead by practising using a condom on their own.

On the plus side, condoms are an extremely effective method of birth-control if used with care. According to some studies, as few as four women in a thousand will become pregnant over a year's continuous use. Other studies show higher failure rates, but this is clearly linked to the commitment or expertise of the users, rather than a failure of the method itself. Some sources suggest using spermicide to increase the effectiveness of the sheath. Making this a necessary condition of condom use, however, increases the 'fuss and bother' attached to the method, and has not been proved to add to its safety. Many sheaths now have their own spermicidal lubrication, and it is likely that this is sufficient.

Condoms provide more than a protection against pregnancy. They are a valuable protection against STDs such as syphilis, trich, gonorrhoea and chlamydia. The last two can both lead to PID. They can protect against herpes lesions and genital warts invading your vagina and cervix, although external sores and infestations from crabs are obviously not ruled out. By preventing the exchange of body fluids, condoms are likely to give some protection against AIDS. Since cervical infection – particularly in young women – is associated with an increased risk of developing pre-cancerous cell changes, it does suggest strongly that barrier contraception may protect against cancer of the cervix.

Condoms can be very useful in other ways. If you and your partner are spontaneous lovers and prone to have intercourse in the morning or just before going out, or *al fresco*, you will know how annoying it can be to 'seep' semen afterwards. Doctors and sexual experts are fond of stigmatizing any woman who finds this inconvenient as a compulsive neurotic with an obsession about hygiene. Such 'experts' have obviously never had to laugh off a tell-tale damp patch.

Condoms are available, free, to both men and women from family planning clinics although not from general practitioners. They are also now on sale at chemists, supermarkets and some cosmetic and fashion stores. They have no health risks or side-effects apart from the occasional allergy or reaction to rubber or to the chemicals used in the lubrication and spermicide. If you or your partner develops an allergy you can use 'allergy' sheaths which are free from lubrication.

## CAP AND DIAPHRAGM

The names cap and diaphragm tend to be used interchangeably but, in fact, they describe two slightly different variations on the same method. This is a device made of rubber that is placed in the vagina and forms a barrier preventing the passage of sperm through the os and into the uterus. The diaphragm is the more popular version. It is a dome of rubber with a rim that contains a coil or strip of metal to make it pliable yet firm. Diaphragms can be from 55 to 100 mm. in diameter. They are designed to lie slanting across the end of the vagina, enclosing the cervix, vaginal vault and part of the anterior or front wall of the vagina. In this position, a correctly fitted diaphragm will be held in place and not be dislodged by love-making. However, since the vagina does 'balloon' during sexual excitement, the device is thought not to be able to provide a consistent barrier. For this reason, professionals advising on the method usually insist that a sperm-killing cream or jelly be used as well. Indeed, diaphragms are often considered to be no more than a way of carrying spermicide to the cervix and holding it there.

A diaphragm is inserted by the woman, or her partner, at any time prior to making love – just before, or several hours in advance. If this is done fairly soon before love-making, spermicidal cream or jelly is spread on the rubber dome which is then squeezed and folded to make it tampon-shaped and -sized. It is then guided into the vagina and pushed up until it unfolds at the top of the vault, covering the cervix. With the middle or index finger, the user checks that the cervix can be felt through the rubber of the dome, showing that the device is in place over it. If the diaphragm is put in ahead of intercourse, spermicide can be left off and added nearer the time of love-making.

Caps are smaller than diaphragms, only 22 to 31 mm. in diameter, and are designed to fit closely over the cervix itself. They stay there by suction and are close-fitting enough to be efficient without necessarily needing spermicides.

Both caps and diaphragms must be left in place for at least six hours after having sex, to give the spermicide a chance to work and to allow normal acidity in the vagina to kill sperm. If you make love a

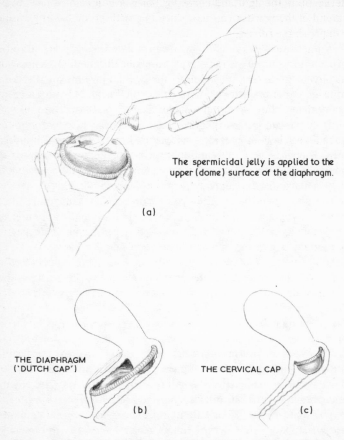

The spermicidal jelly is applied to the upper (dome) surface of the diaphragm.

(a)

THE DIAPHRAGM ('DUTCH CAP')

(b)

THE CERVICAL CAP

(c)

Using a diaphragm or cap: *a* partners applying jelly to a diaphragm; *b* the diaphragm and *c* the cervical cap in place

second or even third time, you are advised to top up your spermicide and to count the six hours before removing your device from the last act of intercourse. To remove a cap, you need to knock the device off the cervix with a fingertip before hooking it out. A diaphragm is drawn out with one or two fingers. Women with short fingers or long vaginas can use a special 'remover' to do this.

After use, the cap or diaphragm is washed in warm water. Before dusting it with powder and storing it in its own container, hold the device up to the light and check for holes or cracks. You need to be careful of the powder you use, since talc with an oil-based perfume can perish the rubber.

Women are often put off trying a cap or diaphragm by the attitudes of doctors or nurses who still largely describe this method as messy or inconvenient. In fact, it is no more messy than love-making itself – a squishy, damp procedure if done with enjoyment. It is no more inconvenient to have to put in a cap or diaphragm than it is to take off your clothes before making love. Used consistently, these two methods have a very low failure rate – as few as three women in a hundred using such a device for a year might become pregnant. Female barrier methods also offer some protection against cervical and pelvic infections and against development of cancer of the cervix.

The disadvantages are that you *do* need to plan ahead or to be confident enough to call for a 'time out' during the preliminaries to love-making, either to put in the device or spermicide. Since we are *not* certain how essential it is to use spermicide, a trial is going on at the moment to compare efficiency rates with and without it, but until the results are known it is better to be safe. Using this method also requires that you are happy about handling yourself intimately, and find it easy. Women with disabilities, or from cultures that require they only touch their genitals with one hand, may find this difficult or may need a partner's co-operation. Diaphragms also have one health risk in that they can increase your chance of developing cystitis or urethritis. This is because the rim can be pressed against delicate tissue by your partner's movements and set up inflammation. Some men find they can feel the device in place, and women can experience a certain loss of sensation. Although the cervix and vaginal vault are not particularly rich in nerve endings, many women can feel – almost subliminally – the rush of sensation as the man ejaculates, and this may trigger their own orgasms.

The muscle tone of the vagina can change over a period of time. Age, or trauma due to a birth, a miscarriage or an abortion, or a loss or gain of weight of more than three kilograms or half a stone can make a cap or diaphragm that did fit suddenly ineffective. After any such change, or every six to twelve months, this should be checked by a doctor or nurse. Since fit *is* so important, and can best be worked out by a trained professional, the initial choice of a vaginal barrier method must be done with the help of a doctor or nurse after a pelvic examination. If you lose or damage your device and have no reason to feel any change has taken place, you can replace it over-the-counter from a chemist. However, they *are* available free from family doctors and clinics, as is a regular supply of spermicides. The NHS idea of how often couples make love can sometimes be at odds with your own experience, so if you use this method you may find you have to supplement your supplies with more bought at a chemist.

## SPONGES

A relatively new variation on a very old theme is the contraceptive sponge. This is a disposable device made of polyurethane foam. Sponges dipped in vinegar or lemon juice have been used as birth control devices from pre-biblical times, but the modern sponge improves on this idea. It is impregnated with a spermicide and is exceptionally absorbent. The device is around 5.5 cm. in diameter and some 2.5 cm. thick. On one side there is a deep dimple, and a loop of material is attached. To use it, you moisten the sponge, to activate the spermicide, and push it high into your vagina, until the dimple rests over the cervix. The sponge must be left in place for six hours after love-making, but it can be put in as much as twenty-four hours beforehand and sex can take place at any time and as often as you like during this period. The device is removed by hooking the loop with a finger and pulling it out. It is then thrown away. Like a condom, sponges are designed for one use only.

The obvious advantages of the sponge are that it is not only free of mess in itself but also soaks up semen – no more sleeping on the damp patch! It can be inserted quite some time before love-making is expected to happen and there are no extra precautions to be remembered. Like a condom, it can be bought from virtually any chemist at a moment's notice. There are no side-effects or health risks. The major disadvantage is that it has a high failure rate of 9 to 25 per cent.

## SPERMICIDES

Spermicides are chemicals that form a barrier to stop and destroy sperm. They come in the form of creams or jellies, aerosol foams, pessaries or film. Creams or jellies may be squeezed from their tubes on to diaphragms. They can also be put into an applicator – a syringe with a blunt nozzle – that is inserted into the vagina: the contents are then pushed out into the vaginal vault. Aerosol foams are used this way as well. Pessaries are a solid gel made in a tampon-like shape, which are pushed up into the vagina and left for a few minutes to melt. The solid film can be inserted into the vagina or draped over the head of the man's penis.

Spermicides not only act on sperm, but also on germs. There is ample evidence that a wide range of STDs, including the AIDS virus, are inactivated by them – particularly by the chemical Nonoxynol-9, which is a major ingredient in most spermicides today. Spermicides also form a barrier protecting against the risk of cancer of the cervix.

Spermicides on their own have a poor record for contraceptive efficiency, although studies disagree on this. An American study, for instance, showed that a large group of well-motivated women had as few as four pregnancies per hundred over a year's use – as good as the IUCD, diaphragm or condom. Other studies suggest a lower efficiency, probably on a par with the sponge. Spermicides, as far as we know, do seem to improve the efficiency of other barrier methods and on their own are certainly better than nothing. They are also effective in cases where you already have a reduced risk of becoming pregnant – during the 'safe' times in your cycle, or as fertility wanes approaching and during the menopause.

Spermicides carry no health risks, although a few women or their partners may experience an allergic reaction to the chemicals used. They are also largely protective against STDs and cancer of the cervix. Doctors and clinics can prescribe them free, or they can be bought over-the-counter without the need for a visit to a doctor or other health professional and do put total control of your contraception into your own hands.

## DOUCHING

Douching means washing out the vagina with a solution of soap and water; water and an acid such as lemon juice, vinegar or a proprietary product or plain water. It can be done as a hygienic action, or as a form of birth-control. It is unnecessary for the former and ineffective as the latter. As already mentioned in Chapter 1 the vagina has its own highly efficient self-cleaning mechanisms, and interfering with these can actually upset the delicate balance of bacteria and natural chemicals in your body and leave you *more* prone to vaginal infection than if you left well alone. Squirting water up into the vagina to wash away sperm is a genuine case of closing the stable door after the horse has gone. Even if you leapt up immediately after your partner's orgasm, by the time the douche has been introduced some sperm will already be in the os.

Douching has other health risks. Passing a solution into the vagina with some pressure risks forcing some up into the uterus, carrying bacteria which are normally kept out of this area. There is thus a risk of PID from the use of this method.

## CONTRACEPTIVE METHODS THAT ARE INDEPENDENT ──── OF LOVE-MAKING ────

There are four methods that are totally separated from the actual act of love: oral contraception, the IUCD, injectable contraception and sterilization.

### ORAL CONTRACEPTION

Oral contraception, or the Pill, has been available in the UK since 1961. It was hailed in the 1960s as 'the contraceptive you can eat', a novel concept in a time of mechanical contraception, and was seen as a major development. It was, but twenty-five years later we are able to see it in a different perspective, warts and all. Rather than being the be-all-and-end-all, oral contraception should be viewed as just one more method to be chosen from a range of equally valid options. The only problem is that too many doctors and scientists and too many users see the Pill as the top of the range – the 'almost ideal' towards which all present and any future methods must aspire. The fact that the Pill is almost 100 per cent effective, almost entirely free from mess and bother and certainly divorced from the sexual act, means that we have set up efficient, mess-free and intercourse-independent contraception as our goal. To many women, this is not actually the point.

Oral contraception comes in two basic types – combined and progestogen-only.

## Combined oral contraception

This consists of a measured daily dose of two hormones – synthetic forms of oestrogen and progestogen. They work by affecting the hypothalamus and pituitary glands and suppressing the hormones that trigger ovulation. As long as these pills are taken regularly, follicles do not ripen in the ovaries and so pregnancy cannot occur.

In the early days of the Pill, quite a high dose of oestrogen was used. Later studies proved that this was associated with health risks and side-effects. Recently, new advances have resulted in very low-dose pills being made available which suit most women and reduce side-effects while still offering complete contraceptive protection.

The most widely used combined pills are presented in packages of twenty-one pills. You take one a day for three weeks, have seven days free of pill-taking and then resume the daily regimen. During the seven days off, you will experience vaginal bleeding. Although the package is marked to show the day or number in the cycle of each pill to aid your memory, each tablet contains the same formula. However, there are combined pills called biphasic or triphasic (two- or three-step) which vary their strength through the cycle. While it would not matter if you got out of sequence on the ordinary combined pill, biphasic or triphasic pills *must* be taken in the correct order.

The bleeding that occurs in the seven pill-free days is not actually a period. Since you do not ovulate while being on the combined pill, the entire normal menstrual cycle is suspended. 'Break-through bleeding' – bleeding or spotting during the three weeks of pill taking – after the first month of starting the pill can be an indication that the dosage is not quite enough for you. The light flow that appears during the pill-free days is, in fact, a 'withdrawal bleed' – a reaction to the change in hormone levels as you stop taking the pills for a short time.

Some women reduce the number of bleeds they have each year by manipulating their pills. If you take four packets end-to-end, only having one week off at the end of a twelve-week period of continuous pill taking, you only have four 'periods' a year. This is actually a healthier and more normal state than having a period each month. The human body is designed by Nature to be pregnant a large part of its life, not to be having thirteen periods a year with only one, two, or three nine-month intervals. Women who suffer from anaemia might benefit from this regimen. You cannot, however, practise this effect if you are on the bi- or triphasic pill. If you want to miss a period for a special event – such as a wedding or a holiday – you can safely do this on your own if you are on the conventional combined pill. Just miss out the seven pill-free days by going from one packet straight on to the next and continue taking that until the end of the twenty-one days. If you are on a bi-or triphasic pill, you can see your doctor or clinic about changing pills for the necessary time. Make sure you go at least a full packet's worth in advance.

The combined pill, whatever its composition, is virtually 100 per cent effective if taken properly. Pregnancies do occur for one of several reasons. Some prescribed or over-the-counter drugs affect digestion and metabolism so that the pill is not absorbed properly and cannot work. Antibiotics such as ampicillin, tetracyclines and rifampicin, most anti-epileptic drugs, some drugs for fungal skin diseases and some tranquillizers, hypnotics, diuretics and analgesics all react in such a way as to prevent the pill giving you contraception. Large doses of vitamin C can also negate the pill. If you lose a pill before it is absorbed, through diarrhoea or vomiting, this too can lead to pregnancy. The worst pills to lose or forget are those at the beginning or end of a packet. Being some twelve hours late taking a pill in the middle of your packet is unlikely to make much difference – but taking the last pill early and the first one of a new packet late may well put you at risk. If pills have been lost or forgotten during the month, you *can* make up for it. If you are less than twelve hours late in taking your pill, simply take it when you remember and do not worry. If you are more than twelve hours late, take one as soon as possible. If you are at the start of a packet, take extra precautions (such as using a condom) for the next seven days. If you are at the end of a packet, start the next packet early, so the missing day becomes day one of the seven-day break.

Alternatively, you could start the next packet immediately and skip the seven-day break, and in that case you do not need to use other precautions. If the missed pill is somewhere in the middle of the packet, use a sheath for fourteen days, even if this extends into your pill-free week and during bleeding.

Some women on the combined pill experience side-effects such as depression, headaches, nausea, breast tenderness, weight increase, tiredness or a lack of sexual interest. If you wear contact lenses, you might find being on the pill can be painful as it can make your eyes slightly dry. The combined pill also increases your risk of suffering thrombosis, high blood-pressure and strokes. For this reason, a doctor would need to check your general health – weight, blood-pressure and other indications – and to ask about your and your family's health before giving you the pill. Any woman who already has some risk factors – has blood relatives with such conditions, is overweight, a smoker or over forty-five – may find her doctor refusing to prescribe this method of contraception.

The main advantage of the combined pill is that it is so easy. Once part of a routine, pill-taking can be convenient and uncomplicated, and your contraceptive measures need never interrupt or interfere with your love-making, however spontaneous and unexpected that might be. The combined pill has some unexpected medical benefits in that it appears to protect you against cancer of the ovaries, endo-metriosis, benign breast tumours, PID and rheumatoid arthritis. It can also reduce anaemia, PMS and painful or heavy periods.

### Progestogen-only pill

Most of the unpleasant side-effects or medically dangerous risks as-sociated with the combined pill are due to its oestrogen content. Women who cannot take this but do want the special convenience of an oral contraceptive may consider the mini-pill. Progestogen-only pills are slightly less effective than combined ones – a failure rate of one or two women per hundred over a year. Instead of simply prevent-ing ovulation, the progestogen in this pill thickens the mucus in the cervix, forming a barrier to sperm. It acts on the endometrium or lining of the womb, so that it is unreceptive to any fertilized egg that tries to embed there. However, progestogen *does* also affect ovulation in many women.

The big difference in mini-pill taking is that the contraceptive effect of this method passes from your body far more quickly. While you can have up to twelve hours' leeway on taking the combined pill, if you are more than three hours late taking your progestogen-only pill you may become pregnant. However, the effect is restored equally quickly, so if you do miss or lose a pill and then resume it, you need only use a barrier method for two days before your pill restores protection. Progestogen-only pills are packaged in groups of twenty-eight or thirty-five and are meant to be taken continuously, even through your monthly bleed.

Periods do come every twenty-eight days or so, but can be erratic and some women find they stop altogether. This may be alarming at first, since you are unsure whether this is a side-effect of the method or if it means that you are pregnant. Women who *do* find the method stops their periods should take heart in that those who continue to have regular bleeds are more likely to become pregnant while using this method than those who stop bleeding. One unfortunate risk that the progestogen-only pill does seem to increase is that of developing an ectopic pregnancy – a pregnancy in the fallopian tubes. If you use this method and develop any pain in the lower belly, especially if you have missed or had a delayed or light period, you should see a doctor at once.

The mini-pill has all the convenience of the combined pill, including help with PMS. It is also suitable for older women and any women barred for medical reasons from taking the combined pill. Oral contraceptives can only be obtained on prescription and in person from a doctor. You can choose whether you see your own family doctor, a doctor at a family planning clinic or indeed any other doctor offering contraceptive advice. This will all be in confidence, and totally free on the NHS.

## INTERUTERINE CONTRACEPTIVE DEVICES

IUCDs are small devices made of plastic and copper that fit inside the uterus. We are not entirely certain how these work. It is thought that the presence of a foreign body in the womb encourages a change in secretion. Inflammatory cells and hormones are produced that discourage fertilized eggs from implanting in the endometrium or lining of the womb. The copper used in IUCDs increases this effect and also acts as a spermicide. It is also likely that the fallopian tubes react, moving the egg down at a rate too quick for fertilization to take place.

The IUCD has to be put in place by a trained and experienced doctor or nurse. This is best done while the woman is menstruating. At this time, the cervix is softened and the os slightly dilated or open. The flow of blood would wash out any bacteria introduced by mistake along with the device. It also masks the slight blood flow that insertion at any other time can trigger, and which may be alarming.

For the insertion of the device, the woman removes her lower clothing and lies on a couch, allowing the doctor a good view. After an initial bi-manual examination, a speculum is inserted. The doctor then takes a 'sound' – a plastic rod is used to measure the length of the uterus. The IUCD is passed into the uterus via an 'introducer' – a hollow rod, pre-set to the measurement established by the sound –

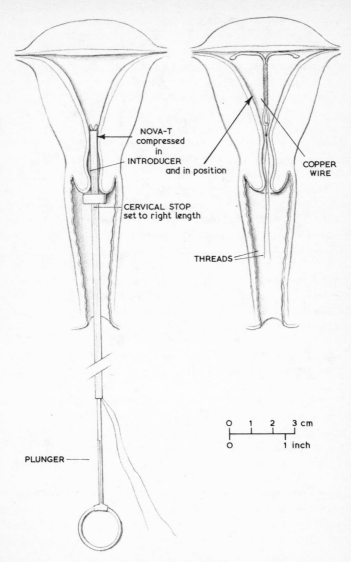

NOVA-T
compressed
in
INTRODUCER
and in position

COPPER
WIRE

CERVICAL STOP
set to right length

THREADS

PLUNGER

0   1   2   3 cm

0           1 inch

Insertion of an IUCD

to deliver the device the right distance inside the body. You may be offered a 'pre-med' or a sedative to help yòu relax during the procedure and the doctor may inject a small amount of local anaesthetic into the cervix.

You might be surprised to find the doctor watching your face rather than your cervix at the last moments of insertion. This is because any pain or shock will show most quickly at this point. If you go white or flinch, the doctor can stop or retreat before the situation becomes more uncomfortable for you. After passing the device into the right position inside the uterus, the introducer is removed, leaving the IUCD open and in place. Threads attached to the end will protrude out of the cervix and these are trimmed to about 1 to 2 cm. long. All you need do in future is to check with an index finger after your period that the threads are still in place, and to have the device changed every two to four years, depending on your age. The younger and more fertile you are, the shorter the effective time-span.

IUCDs can increase the length and heaviness of your periods. They may also be associated with PID. Women with multiple partners, who are more at risk of catching an STD, are not advised to have an IUCD. For this reason, young women who have not settled down or completed their families and who could thus have a greater chance of changing their partners and a greater reason to suffer from being made infertile, may find their doctor refusing to fit this contraceptive device. Women whose wombs have not been stretched by a pregnancy may also find an IUCD painful, as the uterus flexes and contracts and squeezes against the device. This can itself lead to PID or to the device being expelled through the uterine wall into the pelvic cavity – a perforation. Perforations, however, are most likely to happen when the device is put in by an inexperienced doctor, which is why it is really important to see a properly trained doctor who fits IUCDs regularly. The IUCD shares with the progestogen-only pill an increased risk of ectopic pregnancy. It is, however, a very reliable method. Some 99 to 96 per cent of women using it over a year find it protects them from a pregnancy. IUCDs are available free from family doctors and family planning clinics.

## THE INJECTABLE

The 'jab' is an injection of progestogen that works in much the same way as the progestogen-only pill. It does, however, affect ovulation and so is slightly safer. The injection is given into the buttock or sometimes into the shoulder muscle. It should be given within five days of your starting a period, and it lasts for eight to twelve weeks at a time, depending on which type you are given. As with the mini-pill, your periods may become erratic or stop altogether while using this method. Its big advantage is its ease – except for a visit to a doctor every two to three months, the user need do nothing and remember nothing else. However, if you *do* suffer side-effects, such as weight gain, headaches, nausea or depression, you are stuck with them for some time. Also, while your fertility will return to normal fairly quickly after using most other methods, delays of up to eighteen months are fairly common after using the injectable.

Injectables have generally been used by women in particular circumstances – those waiting for a husband's vasectomy to take effect or women who have just had a rubella immunization and so must not become pregnant. It is, however, a first-rate choice for women who cannot keep to a pill-taking routine but who need reliable contraception and find other methods unacceptable. This can include women who have jobs that require they work variable shifts, or women whose home life is erratic. The jab has been the focus of worry and anger from women who feel that it has been used without their consent on those labelled 'inadequate' by their medical advisers. Whether this is true or not, the method remains the *chosen* contraceptive of many. Any doctor can offer it, free on the NHS.

## STERILIZATION

Sterilization is the only permanent method of birth-control. It is a minor operation that makes it theoretically impossible for the man to make the woman pregnant or for the woman herself to become pregnant.

### Male sterilization

Male sterilization or vasectomy is a very quick and easy procedure. So much so, that in some countries it is done by non-medical, specially trained personnel. After a local anaesthetic, a small cut is made in the scrotum or bag holding the testicles. The tubes – the vas deferens – that carry the sperm from their area of production to the outside are pulled into view and cut or blocked. This can take as little as five to ten minutes, and after a short recovery time the man is able to go

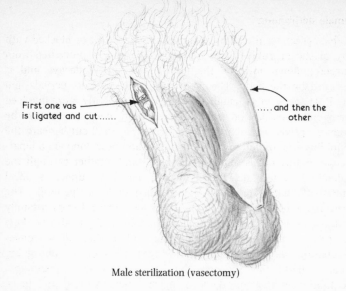

First one vas
is ligated and cut......

.....and then the
other

Male sterilization (vasectomy)

home. The operation has no effect on the man's sexual drive or on sexual intercourse. Since some 98 per cent of the ejaculate is seminal fluid, produced by the prostate and Cowpers Glands further on in the body, neither the man nor his partner could tell by look or by feel that the operation had taken place.

Doctors are now likely to flush out the vas in between the site of the operation and its exit via the urethra. This should expel any sperm left in the tube. However, some can remain, so it is suggested that other precautions are used for a month or so after the operation and sperm samples are then taken to see there are no more viable sperm left. Very rarely, the vas can rejoin themselves, and a vasectomized man can return to being fertile. This is unlikely, however, and not to be banked on. The 'trapped' sperm is reabsorbed harmlessly back into the body. But there is a reaction to vasectomy that means even if the vas is reconstructed, the man may prove to be infertile. The longer the period between sterilization and reversal, the more likely it is that this has happened. Vasectomies are available in hospitals on the NHS after a referral from a family doctor or a doctor at a family planning clinic. Some family doctors even offer them themselves in approved surgeries, and they are also available at private clinics for a fee.

### Female sterilization

In this operation, the fallopian tubes are cut, burnt or blocked with tiny plastic or rubber clips or loops. The egg is prevented from travelling down towards the uterus and simply decays and is absorbed by the body. The menstrual cycle, with its periods and any PMS, goes on as usual. The operation is slightly more involved than male sterilization since the surgeon needs to enter the woman's pelvis. This can be done through a small cut beneath the bikini line – a laparotomy – but is more often now done via a laparoscopy. A tiny cut is made in the navel and another through the abdominal wall. The operation can be done under a local anaesthetic but is more often performed under a 'general'. The operation is obtained free on the NHS after referral from a family doctor or a doctor at a family planning clinic. It can also be done at a private clinic for a fee. Some clinics and hospitals allow women to attend as day-care patients, arriving in the morning and going home at night after the operation. As in the case of vasectomy, sterilization is best considered as a permanent method, not to be tried and then abandoned. Reversal operations can be tricky and have variable results. Sterilization is also a step that should only be seen as a method of contraception. It cannot offer the answer to an ailing marriage or to sexual problems or menstrual difficulties. Indeed, there is some evidence to suggest that some women may find their periods becoming heavier and less regular after this operation.

Since sterilization is almost certainly irrevocable, doctors do ask their patients to be certain before going ahead. You may be asked to attend a counselling session with the doctor or a counsellor to discuss why you have opted for this method, so that the doctor may be reassured that you really understand all aspects of the operation and its results. Although each adult has the right to consent to their own treatment, husbands and wives or stable couples are usually seen together. Neither of you can stop or insist on the procedure for the other one, but if your partner held very different views from you on the subject, it would be irresponsible for the doctor to ignore this situation and not discuss it.

The main advantage of sterilization, of course, is that not only is it hassle-free and separate from love-making, but once chosen you need never consider the risk of pregnancy again.

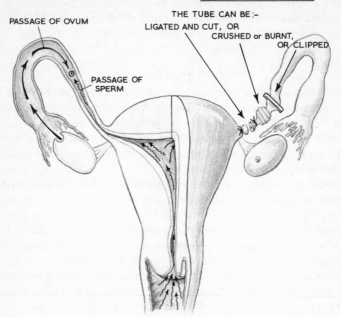

Female sterilization

# CONTRACEPTIVE METHODS
# THAT CAN BE USED AFTER
# —— MAKING LOVE ——

There are two methods of birth-control that can be used in an emergency after unprotected sex has taken place. Both of these take advantage of the fact that Nature itself builds in certain 'fail-safes' in the long journey from follicle and sperm to developed baby. Even if the sperm and egg do meet in the fallopian tube, either may be damaged or aged beyond the point where fertilization is possible. If it is possible, there may still be a reason why the body rejects implantation, or why even after implantation the hormonal cues are not enough to prevent the next menstrual period starting and flushing away the early development. Even later in pregnancy, damage in the foetus or illness in the mother may trigger her body to decide to miscarry. Fertilization may be the beginning of life, but Nature often calls a halt to life before it develops to term. We can make use of this mechanism in post-coital or morning-after contraception, either using the IUCD or a special dose of the combined oral contraceptive pill.

## MORNING-AFTER PILLS

When first used, these consisted of a five-day treatment of oestrogen. This often led to nausea and vomiting. More recently, it was found that a regimen using two tablets of oestrogen and progestogen, followed twelve hours later by another two, is just as efficient and less unpleasant. The treatment must be started within seventy-two hours of sex having taken place.

This is *not* a method to try on your own. For a start, the pills used are far stronger than the ones generally prescribed – they contain 50 mg. of oestrogen, while most used today are of 35, 30 or even 20 mg. Trying to 'double up' to achieve around 100 mg. for each dose means you would only increase the amount of progestogen swallowed as well, and this is likely to lead to vomiting. If you use somebody else's pills, you could also run the risk of finding out too late that you are one of the people who should not be taking such hormones. There is also a risk of their not being efficient. If you use pills because you have had sex around the time of ovulation, but forget that you have also made love earlier in the month, you may, in fact, have become pregnant from the earlier exposure. If you want to use morning-after contraception because you hate the idea of regular pills or do not want to see a doctor about contraception, then use condoms. However, as a one-off, or on the rare occasion, this method is a vital safety net. It is thought that it works by putting your endometrium out of sequence. Instead of being ready to receive a fertilized egg seven days after ovulation, the lining of the womb is hostile and the egg is naturally flushed away without implanting. If you need it, see your own doctor, a doctor at a family planning clinic or one at the casualty or accident ward of your local hospital as soon after the event as possible.

## MORNING-AFTER IUCD

An IUCD can be inserted up to five days or 120 hours after risky intercourse. The earlier it is inserted, the more effective it will be. The method works by altering the state of the endometrium and blocking implantation. The particular advantage of using an IUCD is that it can be left in place to give protection after the emergency is over.

## ─────── WHICH METHOD? ───────

In choosing a method, you need to know not which is the 'best' method, but to work out which one suits *you*. You and your partner need to find out what it is you want most from your contraception. Absolute protection from pregnancy? Total freedom to be spontaneous? A measure of protection from various forms of cancer or sexually transmitted disease? An absence of side-effects or health risks? Freedom from a flow of vaginal secretions afterwards? To use a method efficiently, you need to be comfortable, and any distaste or lingering fears about the choice you have made – or which has been made for you – is likely to end in disaster.

Having made a choice, it is also important to note that you and your circumstances may well change. That being so, what was right for one time may no longer be right for you now. There are times in your life when it is more important than others that you should be free from the fear of pregnancy. There are times when you are dithering over the decision to become pregnant and might welcome the opportunity to let chance or Nature take a hand. As you age, methods that might be unacceptable due to lack of confidence or embarrassment become easy. Methods that might have been risky become safer as your fertility reduces.

Most couples may find a typical contraceptive life-history goes as follows. They could use a condom at first, for protection against STDs and cancer as well as pregnancy. Then they may move on to the Pill for a few years until their first child, using the cap just before a planned pregnancy and the IUCD in the intervals between children. After probable completion of family, they may mix diaphragm or cap, condom and sponge use for a few years before deciding on sterilization. They may keep a supply of condoms and sponges as a back-up in case any of their other methods fail or for *al fresco* use at any time.

Above all, it should be noted that birth control is something that exists to put *you* in control of your body and your life. This starts when you make the effort to find out about the methods available and make it *your* choice of a method that fits in with *your* life, needs, beliefs and tastes.

# CHAPTER 7

# Where Do You Go?

Self-examination is only a small part of self-help Well Woman care. It enables you to keep a running check on your health, and it reminds you constantly that to a certain extent you have a personal responsibility for your own well-being, and the power to affect it. Self-examination can become a part of a range of strategies that might include adding regular exercise to your daily routine, making the effort to prepare a fresh and wholesome diet and avoiding cigarettes and excess alcohol. It might also extend to agitating at your workplace or in your community for local, national or even international initiatives to improve the working and living environment.

Self-help care is also a way of assisting our professional advisers to give us the full benefit of their knowledge and skills. To be fully effective, our own behaviour and the advice or treatment available from the medical profession should dovetail. Neither can operate on its own to keep us fully well. The dilemma facing many of us today is how to get the best out of the professional services available to us. Where we go for help and advice can depend on two factors: what we think we want or need, and what is actually on offer.

At the moment, many of us see Well Woman care as consisting of cervical smears and breast checks. These are the health checks we can most conveniently get from our own general practitioners or family planning clinics. They are usually offered, or we ask for them, when we see a doctor about contraception. In effect, we often present ourselves at the surgery or clinic with an enquiry about our birth-control method, knowing that these checks will be part of the consultation. Women who do not use a method of birth-control – because they have religious convictions, are post-menopausal, gay, have had a hysterectomy or are not in a sexual relationship – often slip through the net. The doctor may forget to ask and we may feel it is irrelevant to us.

It can be difficult to ask for or to find Well Woman care. GPs are often very busy and can give the impression that their time is entirely taken up with people who *need* immediate help – those who are ill. You can easily be made to feel that your enquiries or needs are trivial or unusual, or that you are showing neurotic obsession. Chronic conditions, such as painful periods or PMS, cause most conflict. Doctors tend to hate to admit they are stumped. Rather than say they cannot identify the cause of your problem or help you, some will insist that there is no problem – it is all in your fevered, neurotic and *female* imagination. Some are loath to suggest that the answer to your problem may lie outside their field, or that you might hold the key yourself, and offer the only help they can – tranquillizers, antibiotics and a range of inappropriate chemical treatments that might do more harm than good. Tranquillizers emphatically do not help control PMS and may indeed make it *more* difficult for you to cope with the situation.

Given that Well Woman care is 'holistic' – that is, concerned with the whole person, her lifestyle and environment – any attempt to provide it should ideally take the whole package into account. A doctor or centre offering Well Woman care would go beyond simply making provision for cervical smears and breast checks. Doctors would also give more general health checks – blood-pressure, urine and blood tests would be offered alongside checks on other organs and body functions. In such a centre, counsellors would be on hand to discuss sexual problems, stress, diet and fitness and to help us work out how best to structure our lives in a healthier and more pleasant way. This may even mean helping with financial, educational and employment advice! Books, leaflets and videos would be available to give us more information, and there would be an opportunity to meet other women to discuss these subjects. Screening, counselling, advice, information, discussion and support – all are part of Well Woman care and the ideal Well Woman centre would offer them *all*.

Do such centres exist? At the moment, the answer has to be largely, no. In 1981, the Association of Community Health Councils in England and Wales held a conference to discuss Well Woman centres and to suggest guidelines. Their view was that centres should not only provide a comprehensive screening service, but counselling to cover emotional as well as medical needs, and that such centres should be accessible to all women. There have been several surveys since that conference that shed some light on whether these guidelines are being followed.

The main problem in discovering whether Well Woman centres or services exist is the matter of definition. Jo Richardson, Labour spokesperson for women's rights, carried out a survey of District Health Authorities and Health Boards in 1986. 52 per cent of the Authorities reported that they had Well Woman care provision in around 400 clinics or centres. However, when the evidence was further examined, it showed that 78 per cent of these were based on the medical model of what such a centre should be – that is, they offered breast and cytology screening but very little else. Most had been developed from existing family planning or cervical cytology clinics. Many, indeed, were merely the same old clinic with a new name! 17 per cent could be said to be nearer the holistic or 'whole-person' based model of a centre offering a full range of counselling, advice and support, and only 5 per cent were truly set up on these lines.

Many District Health Authorities (DHAs) resist the idea of setting up such a centre on the grounds that they have few resources and that they are needed in more urgent fields. They may further argue that the GP is the right person to be doing preventative medicine, since he or she already has contact with the patient and access to their medical history. This argument is very apt – the whole point of Well Woman care is that the person wanting to do it or have it done is *not* a 'patient', but in good health. A customer, perhaps, or a client. Both she and her doctor might feel that the GP's services are more appropriately taken up with *ill* people. Holistic health involves a range of care that helps us *stay* well, rather than treating illness symptoms as they come up.

So, what can you do to get what you need? Your local Community Health Council (CHC) can tell you whether there is a Well Woman centre in your area. If so, join it and use their services for your own and your family's benefit. If the centre only offers a small part of the help it could give, there are two routes you can follow. You can suggest to the staff that they broaden their range, and you can find out from the CHC if there is a local campaign to encourage this. CHCs in areas such as Brent in London, Wakefield, Victoria and South Manchester, Calderdale and Waltham Forest have been involved strongly in developing Well Woman centres and in urging their DHAs to appreciate the need for, and to provide, the proper services. If this is not a priority of your own CHC, they will at least know of any local women's groups involved in campaigning for them.

Meanwhile, you can set out to provide yourself with cover, if only on a piecemeal basis. Your own GP may be sympathetic. Some Well Woman centres have indeed been set up by GPs, and yours may be interested in using the surgery or health centre to run such sessions – if he or she is not already trying to do so! Your GP may well be happy to offer regular smear tests and to follow up on results. You should discuss this when you have a smear.

The smear testing procedure is not foolproof. Some four million tests are now being taken annually – the rate increased by 24 per cent between 1979 and 1984. However, deaths were reduced in the same period by only 9 per cent. The main problem is that not all women are offered or persuaded to have a smear, and not all choose to take the opportunity. Even when they do, there can be difficulties. A percentage of samples reach the testing laboratory in an unsuitable condition, and so cannot be tested. In such a case, the return form advises a re-test. However, doctors and their staff may only recall the women at once when an abnormal smear has been reported. Similarly, when a CIN I smear is found, the doctor may not advise you directly of the result, but keep his or her own record and offer you a test in six to twelve months. This is fine if you *do* return. If you change doctors in that interval, the smear test report can be overlooked by the next surgery, unless there is a specific computer recall system in operation that follows your move. Most DHAs *have* put their cervical cytology on computerized records with this mind, but they are by no means universal or complete yet. Most only have the resources to offer a comprehensive call and recall service to women in the highest risk ages, and it may take up to ten years for all age-groups to be included. If your doctor is unable to let you know the results of your test, it is worthwhile discussing whether you can ring or visit the surgery soon after the report would have come in and be told its results.

It is also worth noting that all tests have a percentage of error. False positives *and* false negatives occur. The former is a good reason *not* to panic but to go for follow-up checks and treatment if you are recalled; the latter, an excellent reason to continue your own monitoring and to stand by your instinct if you feel that anything *is* wrong. And to insist on regular screening even if you are not summoned for tests by your local Health Authority.

If your own GP is unable to help with regular screening and there is no local Well Woman centre, you can have this done at a local family planning clinic. You may attend this, even though you do not wish to use birth-control, or wish to get your contraceptive advice and supplies from your GP. Any problems, such as vaginal discharge or cystitis, can be dealt with by a Genito-Urinary – or Special or VD – clinic in your nearest large hospital. You do not need a referral from your own GP to attend these clinics and, if asked, they will keep your visit confidential, although it really is in your best interests for your GP to know about any diagnoses and treatments you have had.

If you are using your GP and/or clinics for screening, you can get your information and support from sources such as local women's groups or specific self-help groups. There are groups which deal with most aspects of women's health from PMS to eating problems and most have regional or local contacts.

You *can* obtain a more comprehensive health check-up, with advice on all areas of your health and behaviour, by going to the private sector. Private health insurance firms, such as BUPA and PPP, run their own centres, as do private hospitals or groups such as the Cromwell in London and the Nuffield Group. For a fee, they will not only do a smear, but also mammography – a breast X-ray. Mammography can spot developing breast lumps long before they can be detected by hand. Blood-pressure, heart-rate, hearing, sight and lung function may all be looked at, and a blood sample taken. A consultation will concentrate on eating habits, sleep patterns and stress, and give advice on improving these or support in maintaining healthy habits. However, since such centres do not wish to antagonize GPs, they prefer or often insist on only sending their full report to the client's own doctor. Private clinics can also often provide women with an invaluable safety net. If you have been advised that a mammography or colposcopy, or treatment such as laser cauterization, is necessary but that there is an unacceptable waiting-list in your area, or no facilities, you may choose to seek these in the private sector.

Some charitable organisations, such as the Marie Stopes Clinic based in London, run Well Woman clinics for a reduced fee. Others, such as the WI, Women in the Community and the Women's National Cancer Control Campaign, have mobile screening units which give free checks. These can be hired by employers or the employees' trade union, and offer a check-up to staff in working hours. In 1987, the WNCCC screened 40,000 women employed by

400 groups as diverse as Tesco, Sainsbury's, Barclay's Bank, the House of Lords, several Civil Service departments, Union and Borough Councils. The WNCCC mobile clinics have also been sponsored by public-spirited companies and charitable bodies to set up shop in town centres or housing estates and offer screening to anyone who asks. These are intended as 'starter' tests to catch women who have never been screened before, so that in the future they can have the confidence to visit their own doctors or local clinics for regular screening.

If you are lucky enough to have a properly functioning Well Woman centre in your vicinity, use it. If you are lucky enough to have a sensible and co-operative GP, willing to set up such a service, give him or her all the support you can, and then use it! If neither is available, cover yourself in any way you can, and give your voice to the local pressure groups who are probably campaigning at this moment for just such a facility.

Our health is something that is far too important to leave to chance, or in other people's hands. We have a right to good health and we have a responsibility to do all in our power to maintain our well-being. As already mentioned, our health is very rarely the result of luck or factors *totally* beyond our control. Once you decide to take control of your own body, you may be surprised by how far your feelings of self-confidence and well-being can take you!

—— CHAPTER 8 ——

# Questions and Answers

*I have an eleven-year-old daughter who has started to develop, although she has not yet had her first period. How old should she be before I suggest she learns how to do self-examination?*

There is no lower or upper age-limit to learning about yourself. Indeed, one could argue that around puberty is an ideal time. Young people are both fascinated and alarmed by the changes that occur in their bodies at puberty. The fascination means that she is likely to explore herself, whether you encourage her or not. The alarm is usually occasioned by lack of knowledge and understanding of what she finds – and guilt at touching herself in a secret and forbidden area. If you were to encourage her explorations, you would be doing her a favour. Many young people are caught unawares by the growth and alterations in appearance of their genital organs and become convinced that this has been brought about by their self-exploration. Girls are often unprepared for signs of physical maturation such as hair growth, the change in shape and size of their genitals, increased vaginal lubrication and periods, and are frightened and disgusted by these. Sanitary protection is often a subject that causes distress. Most girls would like to use tampons, but many are nervous about trying, in case the tampon gets lost inside them, inserting one hurts or usage robs them of their virginity. Being familiar with their own bodies and able to discuss this subject with parents and friends could free adolescence of much of its agony.

*OK, I'm convinced! I know I should get into the habit of examining my breasts, but I keep forgetting to do so in the week following my period. Any suggestions?*

Yes – don't wait until your next period, but do your first check NOW. Turn to page 75 and begin. As you say, doing regular health checks *is* something that should become a habit, and getting into the swing of it is the key. Even if today is not the best day of the month, by beginning now you give yourself no excuse to keep putting it off. You also give yourself the first experience of testing out the shape, texture and appearance of your body, against which to measure future checks. If you find your breasts are lumpy now, but less so after your next period, you will start to learn how *your* body reacts to its monthly cycle. It's also a good idea to do vaginal examinations at various times of the month, so you can learn how your vaginal secretions change throughout this time.

*I read somewhere that it isn't really necessary to have a smear test until you are thirty-five and yet you seem to suggest having one earlier. When is the best age to have a first smear?*

If we had infinite resources in our health services, the answer could be, 'When you become sexually mature or sexually active. Whichever is first.' If we had adequate resources, the answer should be, 'When you become sexually active or at thirty-five years old. Whichever comes first.' As it is, the official line encourages women to wait until they are thirty-five, by only paying doctors a special fee for doing a smear test if their patient is thirty-five or over. This deadline is based on the fact that *most* uterine cancers only occur in women over this age, and then proceed slowly. The problem is that in some women reproductive cancers *are* occurring earlier and *are* proceeding more quickly. For this reason, most doctors are willing to offer their patients the protection of a smear test far earlier. The general feeling is that the right time for your first test is soon after you first have sex.

In economic terms, widespread cervical testing may not make sense when offered to younger women, since the majority do not display abnormalities and a significant proportion of those who do revert to normal without needing treatment. But it makes *individual* sense since, in the vast majority of cases, cervical cancer, if caught at an early stage, can be completely eradicated.

The sensible course, if you are under thirty-five, is to discuss with your doctor whether you feel it necessary to have this test. We do know that various elements add to your risk of developing this disease. These include:

Having early sexual intercourse.
Having an early pregnancy.
Frequent pregnancies.
Exposure to STDs or a sexual partner with a history of them – especially herpes and/or genital warts.
Being a smoker.

If you come into any of these categories, you and your doctor are likely to feel justified in your having your first smear test before you are thirty-five.

*How often should I have a smear test?*

Again, economics play a role in the answer to this question. The official guidelines allow for five-yearly tests after you reach thirty-five. The British Medical Association recommends three-yearly smears, the interval preferred by most doctors. The ideal pattern would be an initial test soon after first intercourse, with another a year later. If both are clear, and in the absence of any worrying symptoms, smears should then be taken every three years. If you have been exposed to herpes or genital warts, or if an abnormality has been diagnosed and successfully treated, smears should subsequently be done at least every year.

*Is self-examination something only women need to do, or should men do their own health checks, too?*

If women are the weaker sex, how come we live on average five to six years longer than men? The only difference, perhaps, is that men carry the greater part of their reproductive organs outside their body, making them easier to handle and examine – an ease which they really should exploit. Men should, indeed, make regular checks on their testicles for suspicious lumps and uncomfortable veins or blockages. Since around 2 per cent of breast cancers are found in *male* breasts, a check on this area once in a while would also not go amiss.

Men probably do check up on themselves more often than women do in the process of handling themselves while urinating or washing. The problem is that many, if they do find anything suspicious, fail to act on the discovery. So we should encourage them to do so.

*When I tried to buy a speculum from a leading high street chemist, they refused to sell me one. They implied that this was because an untrained person could do herself some damage using it. Could I harm myself doing these health checks?*

Obviously any object inserted into a bodily orifice *could* do some damage if you are clumsy or impatient. But how much training does it need? Nobody suggests you need a doctor's or a dentist's advice before being allowed to buy tampons or dental floss, yet both can hurt you if used incorrectly. It could be argued, indeed, that using an instrument on yourself is always going to bear less risk than having one applied by another person. You can feel exactly what is happening and stop at the first twinge of discomfort – something a dentist or doctor is not always able to do. As long as you are careful and scrupulously clean, it is most unlikely that you would hurt yourself with a speculum. What you *will* do is stake a claim on a part of your body that up to now has only been seen and examined by doctors and lovers, and get to know it. I have a feeling that it is this act of taking possession that makes some authorities rather uneasy at the idea of all us women running around brandishing specula!

*Surely encouraging people to poke around inside themselves would create an unhealthy obsession with things that are best left alone?*

There is very little in life that *is* 'best left alone'. Infections and cancer are certainly not in that category. *If* by examining your breasts you found a disease about which you or your doctor could do nothing, and by doing so only gained the misery of knowing what was happening, then I *might* agree. Even when a condition is incurable, however, many people *would* like to know as much as possible and make appropriate adjustments.

The fact is that even cancer is not incurable. If ignored and left, of course, most infections get worse and may then have serious repercussions. But the *earlier* a condition is picked up and the quicker treatment is applied, the better your chances. It is not obsessional to be aware of how you look in good health and to test that awareness regularly. Far from being a misplaced obsession, it is a healthy concern – and one that may not only enhance your life: it could save it.

*I had always thought that only a doctor can really make any sense of the symptoms you suggest we look for. So, what use is self-examination if an ordinary person can't understand what they find, or do anything about it?*

Doctors are not given their abilities by divine decree – they *learn* how to recognize and make sense of symptoms, in exactly the same way as you could learn how to understand your own body. In some cases, you may have an advantage over a doctor. With only one body to check rather than the average GP's list of patients, you have the time and the opportunity to make regular examinations and notice even the smallest deviations from the norm. You don't *have* to understand exactly what is wrong and what to do about it. What you are looking for is anything that tells you concern is justified, so that you can *then* approach your doctor for his or her professional skills. In the case of recurrent conditions, such as thrush and cystitis, you can quickly learn to recognize the symptoms and take your own action, which is often enough. Self-examination is not a treatment in itself, nor is it a replacement for professional help. It is a way of using and enhancing your own awareness and self-understanding so that you can make *better* use of professional abilities.

*My widowed mother has never had a smear test and says that since she is no longer bothered by 'all that' (I think she means sex!), she doesn't need to see her doctor for a smear test or breast examination. Is she right?*

NO. Sexual activity might be at the root of some of the conditions that affect our reproductive organs, but that does not mean that celibacy calls a halt to the development of such problems. Having been sexually active earlier in life, she has *already* increased her risk of developing cancer of the cervix – and that risk often does not emerge as a factor until later in life. Furthermore, the longer she delays a check-up, the more likely it is that any conditions that may have developed will not benefit from treatment.

Some 90 per cent of women who end up with advanced cancer of the cervix have never had a smear test. If you are over thirty-five, whatever your present state, you should have regular smear tests. In fact, it really is a case of swings and roundabouts. Women who have always been celibate or not had children will find their chance of developing breast lumps is greater than their sexually active and parous (having given birth) friends!

*I've been faithful all my life to my husband, and he to me – we were both virgins on our wedding night. My doctor has been on at me for some time to have an intimate check-up, but surely this is not necessary for me?*

You have obviously removed some risk factors by your fidelity. But many reproductive disorders have nothing to do with your sexual behaviour. Furthermore, it isn't a simple case of 'catch this and you will then develop that'. All the elements we have mentioned – early sex, a history of STDs, early pregnancy, your age – are risk factors. If you imagine that you start out with a score of zero, each action adds one point. However, the score that means you personally will develop such a disease may be a different score from anyone else. We just don't know all the factors – the air you breathe, the house you live in, the food you eat, the chemical make-up of the man you sleep with or the genes you inherited from your parents may all make you more, or less, likely to suffer from one of a dozen reproductive conditions without any extra help from the fruits of a casual sexual history. Your doctor knows this, hence the gentle insistence on a precautionary check.

*My older sister belongs to a women's health group and is trying to persuade me to go along too. I'm disabled, so I hardly see the need. After all, I'm most unlikely ever to have a boyfriend, so what's the point?*

Every point. Not all our sexual pleasure comes from shared activities. If you see learning to understand your body and how it works as a means of enhancing your sexual pleasure, then you should see the point of this whether you are in a relationship at the moment or not. The best way of learning how to share your body and its pleasures with someone else is first to do so with yourself. But most important of all, your sexual health is a separate issue from your sexual activity. One may trigger problems in the other, but problems can arise whether you are celibate or not. What may be important for you is to recognize that your sexuality and sexual parts are as beautiful and worthwhile as are anyone else's and that you have as much right to get to know them as anyone else.

Who says that being disabled means you will not have a sex life? It is true that in our society sex is still seen as the exclusive property of the young, the slim, the beautiful and the perfect. Most of us are none of these things, but we are desirable in the eyes and hearts of those who love us. Whether or not you have a relationship often depends on luck and attitude – meeting the person or persons that attract you and are attracted by you, and the ability to like yourself enough to accept that they do too. Self-examination, by helping you learn about yourself, can increase your self-esteem.

*I am disabled and have difficulty in holding items steady. I would like to learn how to examine myself – I've had enough of letting other people take charge of my body – but it would be a problem. Any suggestions?*

You will probably need to apply some forward planning and be persistent to achieve what you want. Leave aside, for the moment, the use of a speculum and concentrate on external exploration. A light and a mirror on a stand are obviously helpful for anyone doing self-examination – they can be set up to shine on your genitals and leave both hands free. For you, they will probably be essential. You may also have to ask for the help of attendants or friends in preparing yourself to have a look. The key is to make it clear that this time *you* are in charge and intend calling the shots. If you can assert yourself to this extent, the fact that you may have to ask someone else to insert and open the speculum may become less important than the fact that it will be *you* who is looking, via the mirror, at what it reveals. Even when people have their hands on you, you can be in control . . . if *you* are the one saying yea or nay.

*I am registered with a GP but haven't seen him for years. I visit a homoeopath for any problems. Now, I would like to have a smear test but I'm worried that I'll get a lot of hassle about my beliefs and I certainly don't want to take any pills.*

Many doctors are now seeing alternative medicine as an area that deserves investigation. Acupuncture, for instance, is practised by many NHS physiotherapists as yet one more valuable addition to the methods available to them. You are most likely to find that your doctor is more interested in the fact that you would like a smear test than in your medical beliefs. No treatment or therapy is compulsory – you would not expect it to be so in homoeopathy, and it isn't in conventional medicine. If your doctor suggests a treatment he or she feels is necessary, it is up to you whether you accept or not. Keeping an open mind is a useful skill for both the doctor *and* the patient, by the way!

*I know I should go to my doctor for a smear test, but since he's a man, I feel very uneasy about it.*

A lot of people do feel shy and embarrassed about showing a part of our bodies we tend to think of as 'private' to a virtual stranger. We are brought up to feel that genitals and breasts are areas that adults should only show to sexual partners, and this makes the doctor/patient relationship fraught and uneasy. You might be nervous that a male doctor will overstep the bounds, or interpret questions or contact as sexual in intent rather than medical. Your concern is understood by the medical profession. For this reason, a doctor will always happily allow you to have a chaperone – another person in the room during a consultation, to keep you company and confirm that nothing untoward happens. You can take a close friend or a spouse, or ask that a nurse be present. If a doctor has no one on hand, you can ask for another appointment or for someone to be brought in – a health visitor, for instance. Alternatively, you can ask for this sort of examination to be done by a woman doctor, if your practice has one, or go to your nearest family planning session that can provide a woman doctor. Some doctors are. also happy for their practice nurses to do these examinations for their patients.

*I find my GP most unhelpful – he just will not listen to my worries and makes me feel awkward and stupid. If I ask any questions, he says I've been reading rubbishy women's-libber magazines and that I shouldn't fill my head with things that don't concern me. I wish I was lucky like my neighbour – hers is marvellous and hands out leaflets and encouragement by the handful!*

If it were a shopkeeper or plumber under discussion, you would know just what to do here. You would vote with your feet by taking your custom from the rude and unhelpful to the polite and keen. Being a patient rather than a customer gives you no fewer rights. You pay for your doctor's service, too, and that gives you the right to demand consideration and expertise. The payment may be invisible and come out of your taxes to make up the salary his Family Practitioners Committee pays, rather than a fee for every consultation, but is still a fee paid by you.

Every patient has the right to choose their doctor and to move from one practice to another without having to give an explanation or to ask for permission to do so. All you need to do is to take your medical card along to the surgery of the doctor you would like to see and ask them to take you on. If their list is full, try another, and if you have any problems write to your local Family Practitioners Committee at the address in your local phone book for their help. If more patients were prepared to do this, those doctors who behave with less consideration would soon find that taking a leaf out of their more helpful colleagues' books would be sensible. There's nothing like voting with your feet to make a point!

*I recently had a smear test and breast examination and everything was apparently normal. However, during the visit the doctor said a few things that puzzled me, but I didn't get round to asking what he meant. In fact, I have quite a few questions that I forgot to ask and I now feel very foolish. Who can answer them for me?*

Your doctor. Most of us find medical consultations stressful and baffling, and forget half of the vital questions we would have liked to ask. The way round this is to make a list beforehand of all the things you would like cleared up. Then if something comes up in the consulting room, the chances are that you will be more able to remember to add it to the list. If not, make a new list afterwards and go back a second time. Your doctor is highly unlikely to want you to be in a state of misery or confusion, and so will be delighted to explain. Most doctors are painfully aware that their patients often 'glaze over' during an examination and that remarks go in one ear and out the other. So they also won't be impatient if at the end of the session you say, 'Could you just go over what you have explained again so that I can get it straight in my mind?' and stop for a better explanation on each item that puzzles you.

*My daughter is fifteen and recently has been diagnosed as a diabetic. She has a marvellous consultant at the local hospital who has encouraged her to learn how to inspect herself and look after her health in many ways. Am I being a bit premature in wondering whether vaginal health checks should be part of this – it hasn't been mentioned so far, so I wonder whether I'm being silly?*

You are not being silly at all. The reason why some doctors dealing with this disorder are reluctant to mention 'intimate' check-ups for someone of your daughter's age has, I believe, more to do with our attitudes to sexuality and teenagers than with any need or lack of need for such checks. As your daughter may have already discovered, thrush is often an early symptom of diabetes and can be a problem if she is having difficulty balancing her blood sugar levels. Diabetic care nowadays quite rightly places enormous emphasis on the diabetic's own responsibility for their health. So adding vaginal checks to the other self-help care your daughter will be learning to apply is only logical. Logic, however, often founders in the face of embarrassment, and some doctors do not even try to suggest such care, in case the teenager cringes in embarrassment and Mum reacts with righteous fury! If you were to suggest that your daughter learns to look after herself in this way, I'm sure her consultant would be only too delighted and relieved.

*I value my privacy, so I'm a bit nervous about having an intimate examination. Can a doctor tell that I've masturbated in the past, or whether or not I'm a virgin?*

We all have a right to privacy, but there are times when some information has to be shared for our own good. You would be foolish, for instance, concealing from your doctor the fact that you had had genital warts, herpes or PID, because all these conditions could affect your future health and the treatment your doctor might offer you. What you have to decide is *why* you wish to conceal information. Are you afraid of moral judgements? Your doctor has no right to make them, and if he or she did, could be justifiably reprimanded by you or a higher authority. Are you afraid of word getting round? Any information known to your doctor is strictly confidential and can't be shared with an outsider.

Strictly speaking, your doctor cannot tell from a cursory examination what your sexual practices are. The hymen can be intact in a sexually experienced woman or stretched, broken or non-existent in a virgin. In the majority of cases, the tattered remnants of a hymen might suggest sexual experience, and women who have given birth will probably be recognizable by such a sign. The shape of the os – the channel through the cervix into the uterus – is also changed by childbirth, from a narrow, round hole to a mouth-like slit. However, the greatest protection to your privacy is not that your doctor cannot tell anything by examining you, but the fact that he or she only *cares* about such information in so far as it contributes to your future health care. As such, it isn't an invasion of privacy or fruit for gossip, but essential medical information.

*All this self-examination appears to be a good idea – but it does seem such hard work.*

So is disco dancing, making love and most things that are worth doing. Putting a little effort into an activity does not make it unpleasant or better left alone. You would find ill health a lot more exhausting and unpleasant!

*I recently had a smear test and now I'm worried. I had gonorrhoea when I was a teenager, but I've never told my husband about this. Will my doctor inform him?*

No. A doctor obviously has an appalling dilemma if asked to treat an existing sexually transmitted disease in one member of a partnership when the other partner is ignorant of the situation. But even in this case, the rules are clear – the doctor must seek to persuade the patient to open discussion but must not him- or herself break confidentiality. In your case, not only is the doctor forbidden from passing on this information, but he or she has no reason to do so. The fact that you had gonorrhoea may have little relevance to the result of your smear test, anyway. But whatever the result, it is between you and your doctor. It is up to you what you pass on to a third party.

*I can see the point of being honest about your sexual past and I'd like to know if any of my fiancé's past experiences would put me at risk. But that means I would have to tell him about my earlier boyfriends – and I'm not sure he would like that.*

We do still suffer from a double standard in our society that makes sexual experience in men acceptable if not desirable, but similar experience in women unacceptable. This is unfair, but undeniable. The problem is that your fiancé's past sexual history *is* relevant to your health, but very few people will accept disclosure of such details as just a matter of giving medical information. So he may reasonably demand that if he comes clean to you, it's only fair that you come clean to him. You and he will have to work out between you whether or not honesty will work for you, or be a source of pain and anger.

There is an alternative. If you both have the same doctor, you can ask that he or she has an honest discussion with the two of you separately and then applies the relevant details to deciding your future health care. The doctor can do this without telling you anything disclosed in confidence. But if there is a reason to suggest, for instance, that you need smear tests, you do not need to know whether this is from your background or your partner's.

*I don't sleep around, but I don't have a current boyfriend. A friend tells me she always carries condoms and would insist on any new contact using one. Is this a good idea?*

No. It's an *essential* one! STDs would appear to be more common now than they were twenty years ago. If you have sex with someone who has already had sexual contact with another – or several others – you have a very real risk of their having contracted an STD and passing it on to you. STDs can be unpleasant. Some can also have long-term, serious effects and at least one can even kill you. Some do their worst damage before alerting you with obvious symptoms, and one – HIV or the AIDS virus – is at present both potentially deadly and incurable.

You simply cannot tell by looking at your sexual partner, or even from open and honest discussion, whether or not he has been exposed to an STD. You *can*, however, largely protect yourself from most STDs, including the AIDS virus, by practising Safe Sex; this means avoiding high-risk sexual acts, one of which is the exchange of body fluids. Using a condom efficiently can help in this.

Carrying – and insisting on any lover using – a condom is also a good test of his sincerity and care. If he refuses, is he really someone with whom you want to share such an intimate experience? If he is prepared to put you at risk of disease rather than compromise his pleasure one iota, what does that say about his attitudes to *your* pleasure, your well-being and your place in the relationship?

### How often should I do a vaginal and breast examination?

The most convenient interval is once a month; either in the week following your period or, if you have passed your menopause, on a particular date that suits you and your memory. Missing a few days or a month is nothing to panic about, but doing this once a month means it becomes a pleasantly unhurried and unworrying routine.

### I've had a total hysterectomy and so no longer have a cervix. Does this mean I no longer need to have smear tests?

You have obviously had the site most prone to develop cancerous changes – your cervix – removed, so a pap or smear test as such is no longer possible. However, your doctor may well want you to continue to have a regular HVS (high vaginal swab). Instead of taking cells from the cervix, this takes a sample from the vaginal vault – the cul-de-sac at the top of the vagina. If your hysterectomy was performed because of a malignancy, keeping a regular check on this area is all the more important. Otherwise an HVS at the same interval as you would otherwise have smear tests is probably sensible. Vaginal cancer *is* far rarer than cervical cancer, you will be glad to know!

### I stopped having periods around three years ago. I was one of the lucky ones and had very few problems with the change. As I had no reason to see my doctor, I've not bothered to have a smear test since then. Are they still necessary for me?

Yes, most certainly. Far from being 'still' necessary, it is at your age they become *most* necessary. The arguments over how often and when women should be given smear tests have focused on the younger age groups because it is now recognized that malignant changes can start early, progress slowly and be totally reversed if treated quickly. But what is often forgotten in all the rhetoric is that the reason the Government guidelines suggest women need only be tested when they reach the age of thirty-five is that most women who develop obvious changes do so *later* in life.

*I'm pregnant at the moment and looking forward to having our first baby in three months' time. I've been doing vaginal self-examination for some years now, so I'm curious as to what I can expect to see after the birth. Will I look the same or will there be changes?*

There will be changes, although they are likely to be less dramatic than you might expect. Working from the outside in, the shape of the vulva might have changed and you may notice the fourchette (the fold formed by your labia minora coming together between your vagina and the perineum – the flat area reaching back to the anus) will have smoothed out. Sometimes this is torn or stretched during childbirth and a natural tear or episiotomy scar may be present. Both labia may be darker in colour than before the birth, and instead of turning from pink to red during sexual excitement, they will turn from red to purple. During sexual excitement, while your labia majora once shrank against your body, they will swell by two or three times.

Your vagina may feel slightly less tight, and the walls will look smoother. The cervix is likely to be cone-shaped instead of oval, and the os instead of being round could now be a narrow slit with distinct upper and lower lips.

Your breasts are likely to be enlarged during lactation but return to their former size afterwards. However, they may feel less firm and have faint stretch marks – red lines just below the surface of the skin that fade to a silvery hue. The nipples will darken from pink to brown.

*What are the relative health risks of methods of contraception? I've been on the Pill for ten years now and I'm worried that this might increase my risks of getting breast cancer.*

The evidence one way or the other on this question is confusing and contradictory. Some studies seem to show a definite link between long-term Pill use *before* having a first pregnancy, and the risk of developing breast tumours. Other studies show nothing of the sort. We are just not sure whether there is a link and, if so, how it works. We are, however, pretty certain that using the Pill protects you from developing ovarian and uterine cancers. This is reassuring on one level, but no consolation if you happen to be one of the women who develop breast cancer.

All methods of birth-control have some drawbacks to their many advantages. The greatest advantage of any method is that it protects against pregnancy – a state that can give you thrush, varicose veins and high blood-pressure. More women become ill or die from being pregnant than from using the Pill or any other method of contraception.

Using the IUCD can enhance your risks of suffering an ectopic pregnancy and of developing PID. The threads appear to provide a path into the womb for bacteria, so that women with multiple partners at risk of infection are even more likely to suffer this complication. Diaphragm use may lead to your suffering cystitis from the hard rim pressing on and irritating the bladder. All in all, the only way to approach contraception and its risks is to weigh up your whole situation and take your choice. For further information on contraception see Chapter 6.

# Useful Addresses

Health Education Authority
Hamilton House
Mabledon Place
London WCIH 9TX
Tel: 01 387 9528

Provides free information and leaflets on a wide range of health topics.

Family Planning Association
27–35 Mortimer Street
London WIN 7RJ
Tel: 01 636 7866

Provides free information and leaflets on many aspects of family planning and reproductive health.

Healthline
Tel: 01 980 4848

Telephone information service on a wide range of health topics.

SPOD
286 Camden Road
London N7 OBJ
Tel: 01 607 8851–2

An association to aid sexual and personal relationships of people with a disability.

Women's Health Concern
Ground Floor Flat
17 Earls Terrace
London W8 6LP
Tel: 01 602 6669

Charity providing advice to women on gynaecological and other health subjects. Publishes books and booklets.

Women's Health Information Centre
52 Featherstone Street
London ECIY 8RT
Tel: 01 251 6580 (10 a.m.–4 p.m. Tuesdays and Thursdays)

National information and resource centre on women's health issues. Contact with self-help groups and publications.

Women's Reproductive Rights Information Centre
52–54 Featherstone Street
London ECIY 8RT
Tel: 01 251 6332

Information and support on reproductive health. Newsletter, support groups and library open to all. Publications list. Open Monday to Friday 10 a.m.–5.30 p.m.

# HELP WITH
## ———— SPECIFIC PROBLEMS ————

Terrence Higgins Trust
BM AIDS
London WC1N 3XX
Tel: 01 833 2971

Registered charity offering
information, advice and help on
AIDS.

BACUP (British Association of
Cancer United Patients)
121–123 Charterhouse Street
London EC1M 6AA
Tel: 01 608 1785

Cancer information service.
Offers telephone counselling and
advice and has information
sheets.

BPAS (British Pregnancy
Advisory Service)
Austy Manor
Wootton Wawen
Solihull
West Midlands B95 6DA
Tel: 05642 3225

Charity offering information,
counselling and practical
assistance and treatment on
pregnancy and abortion,
contraception, infertility and
psychosexual problems. Well
Woman Care. Fees charged.

PAS
(Pregnancy Advisory Service)
13 Charlotte Street
London W1P 1HD
Tel: 01 637 8962

Similar service to BPAS.

One Parent Families
255 Kentish Town Road
London NW5 2LX
Tel: 01 267 1361

Advice and support to parents
concerning legal, financial and
emotional difficulties.

Stepfamily
162 Tenison Road
Cambridge CB1 2DP
Tel: 0223 460312 (office)
0223 460313 (counselling)

Self-help groups for step-parents
and children. Newsletter and information booklets.

Mastectomy Association
26 Harrison Street
Kings Cross
London WC1H 8JG
Tel: 01 837 0908

Information and support before
and after mastectomy.

Pelvic Inflammatory Disease
Group
61 Jenner Road
London N16 7RB

Support group for women
suffering from PID.

Patients Association
Room 33
18 Charing Cross Road
London WC2H 0HR
Tel: 01 240 0671

Help and advice on any question
relating to patient care.

Pre-Menstrual Tension Advisory
Service
PO Box 268
Brighton
East Sussex BN3 1RW
Tel: 0273 771366

Advisory and information service
on PMS, particularly concerned
with diet. Booklets and
information pack. Fees
charged.

Brook Advisory Centres
153a East Street
London SE17 2SD
Tel: 01 708 1234

Free advice, counselling and
practical help for young people
on contraception, pregnancy,
abortion, and sexual problems.
Publications list.

DAWN
Boundary House
91–93 Charterhouse Street
London EC1M 6HR
Tel: 01 250 3284

Information and campaigning
group on women and drugs and
alcohol. Leaflets available.

Alcoholics Anonymous
General Service Office
PO Box 1
Stonebow House
Stonebow
York YO1 2NJ
Tel: 0904 644026

More than 2,000 groups
throughout the UK offering help
to anyone with a drinking
problem.

Al-Anon Family Groups
61 Great Dover Street
London SE1 4YF
Tel: 01 403 0888 (24-hour
service)

Support for relatives and close
friends of problem drinkers. Over
800 groups in the UK.

Endometriosis Society
65 Holmdene Avenue
London SE24 6LD
Tel: 01 737 4764 (evenings)

Support and self-help for
endometriosis sufferers.
Newsletter.

Anorexic Aid
The Priory Centre
11 Priory Road
High Wycombe
Bucks HP13 6SL
Tel: 0494 21431

Self-help group for sufferers from anorexia or bulimia nervosa. Quarterly magazine.

TRANX UK Ltd
25a Masons Avenue
Wealdstone
Harrow
Middlesex HA3 5AH
Tel: 01 427 2065/2827

Advice and support for tranquillizer users. Leaflets.

Relate (National Marriage Guidance)
Herbert Gray College
Little Church Street
Rugby CV21 3AP
Tel: 0788 73241

Counselling for problems in relationships.

Rape Crisis Centre
PO Box 69
London WC1X 9NJ
Tel: 01 278 3956 (office)
01 837 1600 (24-hour counselling)

Counselling, medical and legal help on sexual assault.

Association for Post-Natal Illness
7 Gowan Avenue
London SW6 6RH
Tel: 01 731 4867

Support and advice on post-natal depression. Leaflets.

Post-Abortion Counselling Service
340 Westbourne Park Road
London W11 1EQ
Tel: 01 263 7599

Counselling for women who have had an abortion at any time.

British Association for Counselling
37a Sheep Street
Rugby CB21 3BX
Tel: 0788 78328/9

Information on counselling services.

CAB (Citizens Advice Bureaux)
Myddelton House
115–123 Pentonville Road
London N1 9LS
Tel: 01 833 2181

Free advice on any subject. Local addresses in phone book or library.

Women's Aid Federation
52–54 Featherstone Street
London EC1Y 8RT
Tel: 01 831 8581

Temporary accommodation and
support for women and children
suffering abuse. 120 groups
throughout England.

Parents Anonymous
6–9 Manor Gardens
London N7 6LA
Tel: 01 263 5672/8918
(24-hour service)

Help for parents afraid they may
abuse their children.

OPUS (Organization for Parents
Under Stress)
106 Godstone Road
Whyteleafe
Surrey CR3 OEB
Tel: 01 645 0469

Self-help group for parents under
stress.

Overeaters Anonymous
c/o 6–9 Manor Gardens
London N7 6JY
Tel: 01 868 4109
(answerphone).

Practical help with eating
disorders.

Menopause Collective
c/o WHIC
52 Featherstone Street
London EC1Y 8RT

Information and workshops on
menopause and women's self-
image.

Hysterectomy Support Group
11 Henryson Road
Brockley
London SE4 1HL
Tel: 01 690 5987

Self-help groups for women
having or who have had
hysterectomies.

## HELP WITH PREVENTION,
## —— SELF-TREATMENT AND IMPROVEMENT ——

ASH (Action on Smoking and
Health)
5–11 Mortimer Street
London WIN 7RH
Tel: 01 637 9843/6

Information service and pressure
group on smoking and health.
Free literature.

Association of Community
Health Councils
30 Drayton Park
London N5 1PB
Tel: 01 609 8405

Can put you in touch with your
local CHC.

Marie Stopes House
The Well Woman Centre
108 Whitfield Street
London W1P 6BE
Tel: 01 388 0662

Advice and practical help on all
aspects of women's health. Well
Woman care. Fees charged.

BUPA (British United Provident
Association)
Provident House
Essex Street
London WC2R 3AX
Tel: 01 353 9451

Private health insurance
company which runs fee-
charging screening centres.

PPP (Private Patients Plan)
PPP House
Tunbridge Wells
Kent TN1 2PL
Tel: 0892 40111

See BUPA

Nuffield Hospitals
Aldwych House
71–91 Aldwych
London WC2B 4EE
Tel: 01 404 0601

Private hospitals offering fee-
charging screening services.

Age Concern
Bernard Sunley House
60 Pitcairn Road
Mitcham
Surrey CR4 3LL
Tel: 01 640 5431

Advice, information and
publications on all aspects of
being elderly.

Women's National Cancer
Control Campaign (WNCCC)
1 South Audley Street
London WIY 5DQ
Tel: 01 499 7532–4

Help and advice on prevention
and early detection of breast and
cervical cancer. Leaflets, mobile
clinics.

Royal Association for Disability
and Rehabilitation (RADAR)
25 Mortimer Street
London WIN 8AB
Tel: 01 637 5400

Advice and information on all
aspects of disability. More than
400 local associations. Leaflets.

British Holistic Medical
Association
179 Gloucester Place
London NW1 6DX
Tel: 01 262 5299

Education and information for
doctors and general public on
holistic medicine. Has reading
lists, addresses and leaflets.

Keep Fit Association
16 Upper Woburn Place
London WC1H 0QG

Movement training for women of
all ages. Leaflets and addresses of
local classes.

Sports Council
16 Upper Woburn Place
London WC1H 0QP
Tel: 01 388 1277

Can put you in touch with local
sports centres and activities.

Weight Watchers
11 Fairacres
Dedworth Road
Windsor
Berks SL4 4UY
Tel: 07538 56751

Nationwide network of slimming
clubs. Fees charged.

Slimming Magazine Clubs
9 Kendrick Mews
London SW7 3AG
Tel: 01 225 1711

See Weight Watchers.

Clinic for Cancer Prevention
Advice
6 New Road
Brighton
Sussex BN1 1ZX
Tel: 0273 727213

Advice on health, lifestyle and
exercise. Publications.

Sisters Network
c/o Running Magazine
57–61 Mortimer Street
London WIN 7TD

Help and encouragement for women wanting to start jogging or running. The network will put you in touch with a local 'big sister' who will guide and companion you.

John Bell and Croyden
55 Wigmore Street
London WIH OAU
Tel: OI 935 5555

Can supply a plastic speculum by mail order.

# INDEX

# FOR THE BEST IN PAPERBACKS, LOOK FOR THE

In every corner of the world, on every subject under the sun, Penguin represents quality and variety – the very best in publishing today.

For complete information about books available from Penguin – including Pelicans, Puffins, Peregrines and Penguin Classics – and how to order them, write to us at the appropriate address below. Please note that for copyright reasons the selection of books varies from country to country.

---

**In the United Kingdom:** Please write to *Dept E.P., Penguin Books Ltd, Harmondsworth, Middlesex, UB7 0DA*

If you have any difficulty in obtaining a title, please send your order with the correct money, plus ten per cent for postage and packaging, to *PO Box No 11, West Drayton, Middlesex*

**In the United States:** Please write to *Dept BA, Penguin, 299 Murray Hill Parkway, East Rutherford, New Jersey 07073*

**In Canada:** Please write to *Penguin Books Canada Ltd, 2801 John Street, Markham, Ontario L3R 1B4*

**In Australia:** Please write to the *Marketing Department, Penguin Books Australia Ltd, P.O. Box 257, Ringwood, Victoria 3134*

**In New Zealand:** Please write to the *Marketing Department, Penguin Books (NZ) Ltd, Private Bag, Takapuna, Auckland 9*

**In India:** Please write to *Penguin Overseas Ltd, 706 Eros Apartments, 56 Nehru Place, New Delhi, 110019*

**In Holland:** Please write to *Penguin Books Nederland B.V., Postbus 195, NL–1380AD Weesp, Netherlands*

**In Germany:** Please write to *Penguin Books Ltd, Friedrichstrasse 10–12, D–6000 Frankfurt Main 1, Federal Republic of Germany*

**In Spain:** Please write to *Longman Penguin España, Calle San Nicolas 15, E–28013 Madrid, Spain*

**In France:** Please write to *Penguin Books Ltd, 39 Rue de Montmorency, F-75003, Paris, France*

**In Japan:** Please write to *Longman Penguin Japan Co Ltd, Yamaguchi Building, 2–12–9 Kanda Jimbocho, Chiyoda-Ku, Tokyo 101, Japan*